Sexual Attraction in Therapy

This accessible book offers effective protocol for engaging in better sexual decision-making in clinical practice. It demonstrates that damaging sexual behaviors are often the result of a process in which a clinician progresses towards the crossing of a client–clinician boundary.

Sexual Attraction in Therapy explores state-of-the-art research from a multitude of related fields and includes sage advice on how to recognize personal risk factors, manage arousal, identify counterproductive sexual behaviors, and use self-talk to exit sexual situations. Sexual boundary violations usually follow a much longer insidious process and the book carefully discusses and highlights the warning signs for clinicians, which can develop into sexual predicaments affecting their lives and those of their clients, their workplaces and colleagues, and the reputation of the mental health field. Chapters provide essential guidance so that therapists can monitor progress along the Boundary Violation Cycle and, importantly, create organizations far more resistant to poor sexual decision-making.

This text is an excellent teaching guide for clinicians and treatment professionals who seek therapeutic growth for both clients and themselves. Clinicians will be able to improve their decision-making and prevent themselves from engaging in damaging sexual behaviors, and organizations can redesign their approach to include preventative practices.

Michael Shelton, MS, LPC is a Professional Counselor and faculty member at Jefferson University.

Sexual Attraction in Therapy

Managing Feelings of Desire in Clinical Practice

MICHAEL SHELTON

Routledge
Taylor & Francis Group

NEW YORK AND LONDON

First published 2020
by Routledge
605 Third Avenue, New York, NY 10017

and by Routledge
2 Park Square, Milton Park, Abingdon, Oxon, OX14 4RN

Routledge is an imprint of the Taylor & Francis Group, an informa business

© 2020 Taylor & Francis

Library of Congress Cataloging-in-Publication Data
A catalog record for this title has been requested

ISBN: 978-0-367-20593-5 (hbk)
ISBN: 978-0-367-20596-6 (pbk)
ISBN: 978-0-429-26245-6 (ebk)

Typeset in Avenir and Dante
by Swales & Willis, Exeter, Devon, UK

For Donald and Janice

Contents

Introduction

An Overview of the Problem

Every person employed in the mental health field, whether as a counselor, therapist, psychologist, or social worker, knows that it is never acceptable for a professional to engage in a sexual or romantic relationship with a patient. As part of one's education, training, supervision, and licensure preparation the message that sexual and romantic activity between a practitioner and a patient is censurable and harmful is clearly and repeatedly emphasized. Still, there is a long history of sexual boundary violations; consider some of the pioneers in talk therapy who became romantically involved with clients: Carl Jung, Erich Fromm, Frieda Fromm-Reichmann, Harry Stack Sullivan, and Karen Horney (Alpert & Steinberg, 2017; Blechner, 2014). At the time these incidents were justified as instances of transference and countertransference gone awry or even as true love, and the most severe outcome was professional censure. It was not until the late 1960s that malpractice cases arising from boundary violations began to accrue, and two hallmark cases galvanized the field to action. *Zipkin v Freeman* (1968) determined the defendant had manipulated his patient to become his mistress and leave her husband. More infamous, *Roy v Hartogs* (1975) found a provider utilized sexual intercourse as a treatment technique for the patient's presenting problems, leading to an exacerbation of her mental health concerns.

In the wake of this rising awareness of sexual boundary violations efforts to elucidate the actual extent of the problem were undertaken. As one example, Pope, Levenson, and Schover (1979) found that 12% of male and 3% of female psychotherapists reported sexual contact with their clients. A decade later, Simon (1989), a leader on the topic, estimated that 7%–10% of mental health professionals sexually exploit their patients; however, he stated these figures were likely low due to underreporting. The actual incidence, he proposed could be as high as 25%. Professional associations, state licensing boards, and insurers, taking note of these alarming figures and costly financial settlements to victims, began to promulgate official directives banning this behavior.

Collecting Data

Our understanding of the extent of sexual boundary violations in clinical practice comes about by three methods. First, clinician self-reporting, typically through use of anonymous surveys. Carr, Robinson, Stewart, and Kussin (1991), in an early review of the literature, determined that 7.1% to 10.9% of male therapists and 1.9% to 3.5% of female therapists admitted to engaging in intimate contact with patients. Halter, Brown, and Stone (2007), in their exhaustive review of available literature, remind us that self-reporting likely leads us to underestimate the true prevalence of sexual boundary violations. They concluded that while self-reporting over the last two decades indicates a decline in the incidence of the behavior this may be the result of clinicians becoming more secretive due to fear of sanctions.

A second method of determining the extent of sexual boundary violations is patient disclosure of a past sexual boundary violation to a new clinician as well as clinical awareness of transgressing colleagues. Aforementioned Halter et al. (2007) determined between 22% and 26% of patients report having been sexually involved with a previous therapist to another practitioner and between 38% and 52% of health professionals report knowing of colleagues who were sexually involved with patients. This source of data likely too underestimates the extent of sexual boundary violations. Pope (1994) determined that many clinicians simply do not believe clients when they disclose violations by former professionals. Others are so uncomfortable, confused, or overwhelmed by a client's disclosure that they simply do not act on it. Gartrell, Herman, Olarte, Feldstein, and Localio (1987), for example, surveyed 1423 psychiatrists. 65% reported treating patients who had been sexually involved with previous therapists but only 8% reported these incidents.

Finally, we can look at official complaints made to state licensing boards and/or professional associations. In two early studies, occurring at a time when far fewer states had licensing boards, Herlihy, Healy, Cook, and Hudson (1987) and a follow-up study 5 years later, Neukrug, Healy, and Herlihy (1992), found that the two most common complaints to licensing boards were practicing without a license or other inaccurate representation of qualifications, and having a sexual relationship with a client. The latter study determined that 20% of complaints made to the board were due to the sexual relationships.

Germaine (1997) surveyed state certification boards for addiction counselors and ascertained that the most common complaint involved a sexual relationship with a current client, which comprised 16% of complaints. Neukrug, Milliken, and Walden (2001) surveyed state credentialing boards and found the behavior most often leading to disciplinary action was dual relationships. The authors determined 7% of these dual relationships were of a sexual nature. Boland-Prom, Johnson, and Gunaganti (2015) conducted a study of the types of ethical complaints that resulted in disciplinary actions in the field of social work and found 9.5% were related to sexual relationships. Wilkinson, Smith, and Wimberly (2019), found 9% of ethical complaints to state licensing boards arose from sexual relationships. Finally, Phelan (2007) examined ethical violations leading to expulsion from the major counseling, social work, and psychology associations and found the most common reason for expulsion fell under the category of dual relationships, particularly those of a sexual nature.

Liability insurance providers too track violations since they must pay settlement claims for incidents. In a very recent report, CNA, a leading insurance provider for mental health counselors, determined that engaging in a sexual relationship with a client or a client's family members accounted for 36.4% of all closed claims between the years of 2013 and 2017. The costs associated with these cases are staggering, at an average of $113,642 (Healthcare Providers Service Organization & CNA, 2019).

Using all of the above sources of data, Celenza (2007) estimated the incidence rate of professional sexual boundary violations between professionals in the mental health field and their clients is between 7% and 12%. She also determined that males are overrepresented in these violations and account for 7%–9% while females account for 2%–3%.

Professional Directives

For decades, numerous entities have acknowledged the problem of sexual boundary violations and collectively urged the creation of safeguards against the behavior. State licensing boards are an example. Each state in the United States has its own licensing board that oversees activity in its respective jurisdiction. My state of Pennsylvania, as part of the licensure process, requires petitioners to read and sign an ethical statement, which includes the directive, "Sexual intimacies between a licensed professional counselor and a current client/patient, or an immediate family member of a current client/patient, are prohibited" (State Board of Social Workers, Marriage and Family Therapists and Professional Counselors, n.d.).

Professional associations too dictate that sexual and romantic relationships with clients are unethical. Consider the official pronouncements by the largest professional associations in the field:

- The American Counseling Association – Sexual and/or romantic counselor – client interactions or relationships with current clients, their romantic partners, or their family members are prohibited. This prohibition applies to both in-person and electronic interactions or relationships (American Counseling Association, 2014).
- The National Association of Social Workers – Social workers should under no circumstances engage in sexual activities, inappropriate sexual communications through the use of technology or in person, or sexual contact with current clients, whether such contact is consensual or forced (National Association of Social Workers, 2017).
- The American Psychological Association – Psychologists do not engage in sexual intimacies with current therapy clients/patients (The American Psychological Association, 2017).
- The American Association of Sexuality Educators, Counselors and Therapists – The Certified member practicing education, counseling or therapy shall not engage, attempt to engage or offer to engage a potential, current, or former consumer in sexual behavior whether the consumer consents to such behavior or not (The American Association of Sexuality Educators, Counselors and Therapists, 2014).
- The Association for Addiction Professionals – Addiction Professionals shall not engage in any form of sexual or romantic relationship with any current or former client, nor accept as a client anyone with whom they have engaged in a romantic, sexual, social, or familial relationship. This prohibition includes in-person and electronic interactions and/or relationships (Association for Addiction Professionals, 2016).
- The American Association for Marriage and Family Therapy – Sexual intimacy with current clients or with known members of the client's family system is prohibited (American Association for Marriage and Family Therapy, 2015).

Additionally, an increasing number of states have criminalized sexual activity between mental health professionals and patients. California law, as one example, makes it a crime for a therapist to have sexual contact with a patient. Finally, employers have policies that inform employees that romantic and sexual relationships with clients are prohibited and grounds for termination.

As described above, insurance providers, state licensing boards, professional associations, workplaces, and increasingly the criminal justice system condemn sexual boundary violations. Still, these violations continue to occur.

Damaging Consequences

If the existence of professional directives and ethical statements is not sufficient to deter engagement in a sexual boundary violation, knowledge and even fear of consequences should theoretically be adequate discouragement. Once a sexual boundary violation occurs, the involved clinician must engage in offensive machinations to avoid detection, which in themselves are exhausting. For example, a professional must manage the reactions of the client in order to prevent the latter disclosing the incident; this often includes conspiring with the client to maintain secrecy. Additionally, there is a continued need to keep others from learning about the violation, which requires manipulation of the environment as well as friends, colleagues, and family. These measures complicate the already overwhelming psychological repercussions that frequently follow sexual boundary violations, such as guilt, remorse, and fear.

If and when a sexual violation is made public catastrophic consequences befall professionals engaging in the behavior, including:

- loss of career;
- loss of licensure;
- loss of family, friends, and professional colleagues;
- expulsion from professional organizations;
- financial penalties; and
- civil and criminal lawsuits.

Sexual boundary violations impact not only the involved clinician but also the organization in which they practice. From an organizational perspective, the unearthing of sexual contact between a staff member and a client leads not only to lawsuits, police and governmental investigations, bad press, financial costs, and the dismissal of once-valued staff members but also to institutional trauma. Pervasive denial, helplessness, anger, and guilt form a toxic environment infiltrating the lives of all employees, which leaks into the treatment milieu. Brown (1997) compellingly argues that in the aftermath of a sexual boundary violation, in which the sole focus is on the victim, the reactions of colleagues and supervisors, often feeling betrayed and aghast, are inadvertently disregarded. Too often the transgressing clinician is terminated and disappears completely from their lives and staff end up coping on their own. In sum, a sexual boundary violation leads to an institutional crisis and can have long-term traumatic effects (Honig & Barron, 2013).

Finally (the topic amassing the most research), sexual boundary violations do considerable and often lasting damage to clients. Whether the violation is a singular instance or evolves into an ongoing sexual and/or romantic relationship, frequent sequelae are noted (Luepker, 1999; Pope, 1994; Tschan, 2014; Wohlberg, 1999) which can occur quickly or have a delayed onset:

- guilt and self-blame;
- ambivalence about seeing another professional and not trusting themselves to evaluate and select a subsequent provider;
- mental health disorders and symptoms, particularly posttraumatic stress disorder, major depressive disorder, suicidality, and/or substance misuse;
- resurgence of presenting problem(s);
- disrupted relationships;
- disruptions in work or earning potential;
- sexual confusion;
- relationship difficulties; and
- boundary disturbances.

Celenza (2007), a leader in the field, concludes that the damage of boundary violations does not result solely from sexual activity but rather through betrayal of trust, demands for secrecy, reversal of roles, and the abandonment of therapeutic aims. Tschan (2014) defines sexual boundary violations as a "relational crime" since mental health professionals are frequently significant attachment figures for patients; as such, a sexual boundary violation is traumatic. As mentioned earlier, when disclosing to a subsequent clinician many patients are met with disbelief, the impact of the violation is minimized, and they are held as responsible or partially responsible for the act; these responses in themselves are re-traumatizing.

When added to the directives and ethical requirements of licensing boards, professional associations, and workplaces, the noted consequences for clients, organizations, and professionals themselves should ideally act as defenses against sexual boundary violations. Still, they occur. Pope, Keith-Spiegel, and Tabachnick (1986) concluded that reliance on sanctions and fear of consequences has not proven particularly effective in stemming sexual boundary violations.

Parallel Efforts at Prevention

Reducing the prevalence of inappropriate, unethical, and damaging sexual activity is obviously not the sole purview of the mental health field, and the recent spate of high-profile-incidents and media investigations into varied disciplines indicates how widespread the behavior actually is. Several recent meta-analyses and research reviews regarding sexual harassment and sexual assault in the workplace, on college campuses, and within the military offer the mental health treatment field guidance as how to tackle the problem. Efforts at ending inappropriate behavior in these three domains freely borrow from one another, and similarities are noted.

First, the workplace, the military, and universities have moved away from the "bad apple" hypothesis, postulating that the majority of unwanted sexual behavior in these settings is the result of a few sociopathic or highly dangerous individuals. All acknowledge the need to screen for such applicants and to remove them as quickly as possible but also admit that the problem is far more common than the machinations of this relatively small group could account for. In short, individuals with no seeming predisposing factors engage in sexual behaviors antithetical to a discipline or workplace's mission. The mental health field in contrast continues to espouse confidence in the false notion that the majority of sexual boundary violations are the result of a few predatory individuals.

Second, prevention efforts require education that must be comprehensive and ongoing. A one-time and/or brief training is rarely successful. Consider the recommendations of Vladutiu, Martin, and Macy (2011) in their literature review of university-based sexual violence prevention program: trainings should focus on behavioral intent, rape awareness, rape knowledge, rape empathy, and rape myth acceptance for both genders. A later literature review by the Johns Hopkins Center for Injury Research and Policy (2018) also determined the importance of a broad approach, including topics such as rape myths, gender norms, statistics on university based sexual assaults, communication skills, and physical resistance trainings. Regarding the United States military, Turchik and Wilson (2010) reviewed literature and determined that changing normative views about sex and gender is necessary for reducing risk of sexual assault. In all, a prevention program must comprehensively tackle a litany of controversial and uncomfortable topics. Compare this to the current approach in the mental health field, which does not require mandatory training on the topic at all; it is instead interpolated into general ethics trainings. The topic may be partitioned into a mere 10–15 minutes (or less) out of a 3-hour ethics training.

Third, other disciplines and workplaces in general note the importance of bystander participation, in which witnesses such as co-workers intervene to stop inappropriate sexual behavior, protect the victim, and report it to authorities. Universities and the military promote this practice, and its importance is increasingly recognized for workplace sexual harassment prevention. While the mental health field too promotes collegial monitoring and support, such as in burnout prevention efforts, its endeavors in using colleagues to intervene before an irreversible sexual violation occurs are underutilized. Studies that will be addressed later in this text find that colleagues often note subtle changes in colleagues engaging in sexual boundary violations but dismiss them as unimportant. They also have intense ambivalence reporting suspicions to those higher in authority, such as a supervisor or licensing board. Also, the overwhelming majority of treatment agencies do not enlist the help of another important bystander group: clients. This latter group often has uncanny insight into the inner workings of an agency, and they might detect the misbehaviors of staff quicker than other employees.

Finally, all prevention efforts note the importance of organizational change. A 2007 meta-analysis of antecedents of workplace sexual harassment determined organizational culture had the largest effect size of any variable in the review (Willness, Steel, & Lee, 2007). An organizational culture that is consistently civil, fair, transparent, and compassionate influences employees' compliance with written policy. At present, mental health agencies, and the field in general, underestimate the power of organizational influences, which truly do make it more or less likely that sexual boundary violations will occur. They instead hold to the belief that written policy condemning the behavior should suffice and that organizational policy plays no role in their occurrences.

In spite of the commonality of efforts by employers, the military, and universities in reducing inappropriate sexual behavior, there are two notable differences when considering their use in the mental health field. First, the major focus of workplace, military, and university efforts is reduction of sexual harassment and sexual violence; in contrast, the overwhelming majority of sexual boundary violations in mental health practice are not violent acts or even harassment; they are instead the behaviors of clinicians who have become romantically attracted to clients. In many cases, the professional and client report falling in love with each other; Somer and Saadon (1999) found the majority (82%) of clients in their study described past sexual engagement with a therapist as a romantic affair. Patients are often naively complicit in maintaining the secrecy surrounding the changes in a therapeutic relationship. Second, therapy takes place in a private space in which intimacy, empathy, and exploration of relationship dynamics is the norm; in none of the other milieus are these stated or even expected goals. The therapy process is thus by its very nature a risk for development of attraction and arousal, or in the words of Schwartz and Olds (2002), "[P]sychotherapy is a setup for boundary violations" (p.484). This is explored in the next chapter.

A Preview of the Text

This text targets clinicians and other support staff in the mental health field and examines why so many of our colleagues – smart people dedicated to the best interests of their clients – nonetheless find themselves mismanaging romantic attraction and sexual arousal in clinical settings. While the current chapter has enumerated the numerous consequences that follow a sexual boundary violation as well as existing preventative measures, the knowledge of which still does not eradicate the behavior, the majority of the remainder of the text focuses on a process of arousal and attraction in therapy, which perniciously subverts and frequently overwhelms our logic and long-term perspective taking. Chapter 1 focuses on the risks inherent in therapy, an interaction between two people that requires interpersonal intimacy and connection for success but which then also lays the foundation for possible boundary crossings. The same chapter also offers an overview of the six pillars of prevention, recommendations that build upon existing protocol but which fairly apportion responsibilities and obligations to all involved parties, including clinicians, universities and colleges, licensing and certification boards, professional associations, employers, supervisors, insurance providers, and the legal system.

Chapters 2 through 8 elucidate the Boundary Violation Cycle, a process model describing sexual and romantic involvement between mental health professionals and their clients/patients as a cycle composed of seven stages. Readers will identify their own risk and vulnerability factors and of no minor importance learn that risk fluctuates; it is not a static and lifelong predisposition. Readers will gain an understanding of the influence of fantasy, which is indeed the gateway to a boundary violation; sexual activity leading to untoward consequences is almost always preceded by fantasy. They will identify the power of self-talk and distorted thinking, which propel a professional deeper into sexually alarming behaviors. So too will they learn of two prevailing models – the psychodynamic perspective and the Good Lives Model – which conclude unconscious and latent psychological forces influence sexual decision-making. They will recognize the role of non-sexual boundary crossings as preliminary steps leading to the culminating event of an outright violation. Finally, readers will discover the likely outcomes – both short- and long-term – of professional and client sexual and romantic relationships for both parties.

Chapters 9 and 10 expand the discussion beyond the singular sphere of the professional to include education, ongoing training, supervision, and workplace dynamics, all of which are components of the aforementioned six pillars of prevention and necessitate the involvement of all involved parties described earlier. Finally, in Chapter 11, this text examines the controversial concept of rehabilitation of transgressing clinicians.

In sum, this book posits an accurate reframing of sexual boundary violations; it is not that they are the willful acts of dissolute clinicians but rather an unfortunate outcome for those who did not have the knowledge and support needed to traverse an unfortunately common occupational hazard.

Conclusions

Sexual boundary violations have catastrophic outcomes for clinicians, clients, and organizations. Every major mental health association strictly forbids the behavior; licensing and certification boards similarly prohibit sexual activity with clients. Regardless, these violations have long been noted in the mental health treatment field and continue today. Early research focused on predatory clinicians, those who are repeat offenders and must be removed from the field, and it was long thought that they engaged in the majority of sexual boundary violations. While their presence is still noted, it is now known that the majority of violations are not the result of predatory machinations but instead the behavior of clinicians lacking antisocial intent. In reality, sexual boundary violations transgressors are clinicians very much like you and I who are in the field to foster positive change, personal growth, and possibly even social justice.

Current preventive measures will need to be augmented and a beginning direction is to examine the strengths and limitations of approaches used in other domains. Borrowing from other professional fields' efforts at reducing sexual harassment and sexual violence, we find that enhanced education, organization and systems' modifications, and bystander involvement are core recommendations that the mental health field can build upon. Still, in spite of the commonality of efforts by employers, the military, and universities in reducing sexual assault and sexual harassment, there are two differences when considering their transfer to the mental health field: (1) the overwhelming majority of sexual boundary violations arise when clinicians become romantically attracted to clients; and (2) therapy takes place in a private space in which intimacy, empathy, and exploration of relationship dynamics are the norm. In none of the other domains are these stated or expected goals.

Summary

- It is never acceptable for mental health practitioners to become sexually and romantically involved with clients. This directive is recognized and codified by all mental health associations and licensing entities.
- Engagement in a sexual boundary violation leads to catastrophic consequences for professionals, clients, and organizations.
- Insurance providers, state licensing and certification boards, and professional associations report sexual boundary violations are one of the most common formal complaints made against practitioners.
- Workplaces in general, college campuses, and the military have created methods of reducing sexual harassment and sexual violence, some of which are applicable to the mental health field:

  - retiring the once common belief that these behaviors are the result of "bad apples," or in other words, sociopathic individuals inadvertently hired into an organization;
  - prevention efforts require education that must be comprehensive and ongoing;
  - increasing bystander participation and
  - organizational culture changes.

- The overwhelming majority of sexual boundary violations arise from clinicians who have become romantically attracted to clients.

References

Alpert, J. L., & Steinberg, A. L. (2017). Sexual boundary violations: A century of violations and a time to analyze. *Psychoanalytic Psychology, 34*(2), 144–150.

American Association for Marriage and Family Therapy. (2015). *Code of ethics.* Alexandria, Virginia: Author.

American Association of Sexuality Educators, Counselors and Therapists. (2014). *Code of ethics & conduct for AASECT certified member.* Chicago, IL: Author.

American Counseling Association. (2014). *2014 ACA code of ethics*. Alexandria, Virginia: Author.

The American Psychological Association. (2017). *Ethical principles of psychologists and code of conduct*. Washington, DC: Author.

Association for Addiction Professionals. (2016). *Code of ethics*. Alexandria, Virginia: Author.

Blechner, M. J. (2014). Dissociation among psychoanalysts about sexual boundary violations. *Contemporary Psychoanalysis, 50*(1–2), 23–33.

Boland-Prom, K., Johnson, J., & Gunaganti, G. S. (2015). Sanctioning patterns of social work licensing boards, 2000–2009. *Journal of Human Behavior in the Social Environment, 25*(2), 126–136.

Brown, L. S. (1997). Remediation, amends, or denial?. *Professional Psychology: Research and Practice, 28*(3), 297–299.

Carr, M. L., Robinson, G. E., Stewart, D. E., & Kussin, D. (1991). A survey of Canadian psychiatric residents regarding resident-educator sexual contact. *American Journal of Psychiatry, 148*(2), 216–220.

Celenza, A. (2007). *Sexual boundary violations*. Lanham, Maryland: Jason Aronson.

Gartrell, N., Herman, J., Olarte, S., Feldstein, M., & Localio, R. (1987). Reporting practices of psychiatrists who knew of sexual misconduct by colleagues. American. *Journal of Orthopsychiatry, 57*(2), 287–295.

Germaine, J. S. (1997). Ethical practices of certified addiction counselors: A national survey of state certification boards. *Alcoholism Treatment Quarterly, 15*(2), 63–72.

Halter, M., Brown, H., & Stone, J. (2007). Sexual boundary violations by health professionals–An overview of the published empirical literature. Council for Healthcare Regulatory Excellence.

Healthcare Providers Service Organization & CNA. (2019). *Counselor spotlight: Boundaries*. Fort Washington, PA: Author.

Herlihy, B., Healy, M., Cook, E. P., & Hudson, P. (1987). Ethical practices of licensed professional counselors: A survey of state licensing boards. *Counselor Education and Supervision, 27*(1), 69–76.

Honig, R. G., & Barron, J. W. (2013). Restoring institutional integrity in the wake of sexual boundary violations: A case study. *Journal of the American Psychoanalytic Association, 61*(5), 897–924.

Johns Hopkins Center for Injury Research and Policy. (2018). *A public health approach to reducing sexual assault: A report for college campuses*. Baltimore, MD: Johns Hopkins Bloomberg School of Public Health.

Luepker, E. T. (1999). Effects of practitioners' sexual misconduct: A follow-up study. *Journal of the American Academy of Psychiatry and the Law Online, 27*(1), 51–63.

National Association of Social Workers. (2017). *National association of social workers code of ethics*. Washington, DC: Author.

Neukrug, E., Milliken, T., & Walden, S. (2001). Ethical complaints made against credentialed counselors: An updated survey of state licensing boards. *Counselor Education and Supervision, 41*(1), 57–70.

Neukrug, E. S., Healy, M., & Herlihy, B. (1992). Ethical practices of licensed professional counselors: An updated survey of state licensing boards. *Counselor Education and Supervision, 32*(2), 130–141.

Phelan, J. E. (2007). Membership expulsions for ethical violations from major counseling, psychology, and social work organizations in the United States: A 10-year analysis. *Psychological Reports, 101*(1), 145–152.

Pope, K. S. (1994). *Sexual involvement with therapists.* Washington, DC: American Psychological Association.

Pope, K. S., Keith-Spiegel, P., & Tabachnick, B. G. (1986). Sexual attraction to clients: The human therapist and the (sometimes) inhuman training system. *American Psychologist, 41*(2), 147–158.

Pope, K. S., Levenson, H., & Schover, L. R. (1979). Sexual intimacy in psychology training: Results and implications of a national survey. *American Psychologist, 34*(8), 682–689.

Schwartz, R. S., & Olds, J. (2002). A phenomenology of closeness and its application to sexual boundary violations: A framework for therapists in training. *American Journal of Psychotherapy, 56*(4), 480–493.

Simon, R. I. (1989). Sexual exploitation of patients: How it begins before it happens. *Psychiatric Annals, 19*(2), 104–112.

Somer, E., & Saadon, M. (1999). Therapist-client sex: Clients' retrospective reports. *Professional Psychology: Research and Practice, 30*(5), 504–509.

State Board of Social Workers, Marriage and Family Therapists and Professional Counselors. (n.d.). *Licensure of professional counselors.* Harrisburg, PA: Pennsylvania Department of State.

Tschan, W. (2014). *Professional sexual misconduct in institutions: Causes and consequences, prevention and intervention.* Boston: Hogrefe Publishing.

Turchik, J. A., & Wilson, S. M. (2010). Sexual assault in the US military: A review of the literature and recommendations for the future. *Aggression and Violent Behavior, 15*(4), 267–277.

Vladutiu, C. J., Martin, S. L., & Macy, R. J. (2011). College-or university-based sexual assault prevention programs: A review of program outcomes, characteristics, and recommendations. *Trauma, Violence, & Abuse, 12*(2), 67–86.

Wilkinson, T., Smith, D., & Wimberly, R. (2019). Trends in ethical complaints leading to professional counseling licensing boards disciplinary actions. *Journal of Counseling & Development, 97*(1), 98–104.

Willness, C. R., Steel, P., & Lee, K. (2007). A meta-analysis of the antecedents and consequences of workplace sexual harassment. *Personnel Psychology, 60*(1), 127–162.

Wohlberg, J. W. (1999). Treatment subsequent to abuse by a mental health professional: The victim's perspective of what works and what doesn't. *Journal of Sex Education and Therapy, 24*(4), 252–261.

A Roadmap for Navigating the Risks of Therapy

1

In 1989, Robert Simon's seminal article "Sexual Exploitation of Patients: How it Begins Before It Happens" was published in *Psychiatric Annals*. The author concluded sexual boundary violations were not sudden events but rather the results of a gradual and imperceptible process, and he offered the following vignette to illustrate his contention:

> A 48-year-old male therapist began individual insight psychotherapy of a 29-year-old woman who was attractive, divorced, and depressed. The psychotherapist recently had concluded a bitter divorce after 20 years of marriage. For about six months, the therapy progressed with treatment boundaries intact. Then, gradual incursions began. The therapist and patient began to address each other by their first names. The tenor of the therapeutic sessions increasingly became more social with mutual sharing of experiences. For example, on one occasion, the psychiatrist talked about his divorce and his loneliness. The patient responded by describing the various social functions available to divorcees. At the beginning of treatment, sessions were originally terminated in a verbally appropriate manner. However, over time, a handshake at the end of the session progressed to a hug. Initially, the hugs were perfunctory, but therapist and patient began to linger in their termination embraces. In due course, the therapy sessions were rescheduled for the end of the day. Before long, therapist and patient occasionally dined together. Movie dates followed where hand-holding and kissing took place. Eventually a sexual relationship "happened."

(pp. 105–106)

Now, more than three decades later, the same step-wise progression from therapy to sex, built upon what Simon calls a "culmination of many earlier incursions into the treatment process" (p. 106), occurs in current cases of sexual boundary violations. The above example could be easily modified to fit the modern age with inclusion of a sentence about texting and social media as conduits of communication between sessions by both professional and patient. Other than rape in a therapy context – a rare occurrence – sexual boundary violations are the end result of an extended process, whether the involved professional is a psychologist, counselor, therapist, or social worker.

Simon and those that followed determined that there are key features of therapy that facilitate the progression from well-intentioned professional therapeutic work to a sexual boundary violation. These characteristics are so common that they led Honig and Barron (Honig and Barron, 2013) to conclude that for those in the mental health treatment field "boundary violations is a shared occupational hazard" (p. 901).

The Inherent Risks of Therapy

Sexual attraction and arousal are parts of the human condition and will inevitably find their way into the consulting room. This is to be expected and not a need for embarrassment. Neither should they be ignored; as such, learning how to manage arousal and attraction is a core theme of this text.

Attraction and arousal in clinical settings tends to manifest in five ways, as illustrated in Figure 1.1. While practitioners will agree that flirtation, sexual activity, and romantic relationships with clients are clearly wrong, this text will show that even fantasies and preferential treatment can have consequences.

What about the mental health treatment field leads to the shared occupational hazard of boundary violations? First, and above all else, a therapeutic relationship is a unique form of personal interaction that fosters attraction and arousal. According to Schwartz and Olds (2002), there are six reasons for this common outcome.

1. Patients often begin treatment when other relationships in their lives are dissatisfying or dysfunctional. As such, mental health professionals enter a client's life when the latter are most susceptible to attraction to a person who genuinely cares about them.
2. Mental health practitioners experience undulations in their own relationships, including romantic relationships, and need for intimacy

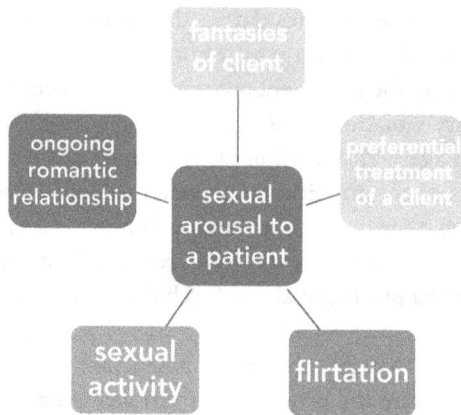

Figure 1.1 The Manifestations of Sexual Arousal in Clinical Settings

themselves; when a therapist is lonely or romantically discontented there will always be appealing and willing patients who could satisfy these desires.

3. Unconditional positive regard, while a recognized crucial ingredient for treatment, paradoxically increases risk for attraction; according to the authors, "The degree of unwavering attentiveness to the patient's thoughts and feelings, to the nuances of the patient's words and gestures is not likely to be matched by the best of lovers or friends over the long haul. The fact that the therapist only sustains that selfless attention over a 50-minute session is too often neglected by both participants" (Schwartz and Olds 2002, pp. 485–486).

4. Therapy aims for ever-increasing levels of intimacy. Even cognitive therapy, an approach not traditionally thought of as entailing profound intimacy, enjoins clients to move beyond an exploration of overt behaviors to underlying automatic thoughts and finally onto their unspoken and implicit core beliefs. Therapy is a progressively intimate experience.

5. Limited self-disclosure by practitioners leads some patients to an extended idealization of them; they never have the opportunity to see the deficits, flaws, and frustrating aspects of a mental health worker's personality that is so readily apparent to their romantic partners, friends, and children.

6. Treatment is conducted without witnesses. Not only does this lead to a lack of surveillance as to what is actually happening behind closed doors in sessions, it also leads to emotional deprivation in existing relationships. Professionals, due to confidentiality laws, are unable to share major

portions of their lives with loved ones, and clients, in turn, withhold their most intimate thoughts and feelings from others in their lives, which are only revealed in therapy sessions. This secrecy prevents concerned others from recognizing that a therapeutic relationship is devolving into boundary violations. According to Schwartz and Olds (2002),

> "Not only is the connection between therapist and patient hidden away from the potentially beneficial gaze of others who care about the patient. The patient's relationships with these others are devitalized by siphoning off from them the patient's most heart-felt concerns. When what is most vivid in our lives is not shared with those we love, our connection with those we love becomes impoverished. That impoverishment is a serious concern for patients and therapists alike. When we live a significant part of our lives without witnesses, we deprive ourselves of more than just a policing presence ... Psychotherapy is a relationship uniquely designed to maximize the experience of interpersonal "flow" within it, while simultaneously insulating both participants from the scrutiny and jealousy of lovers and friends that might act as natural breaks on progressive intimacy.
>
> (p. 490)

Psychological Risks

All clinicians at some point in their career will experience sexual fantasies or sexual attraction towards a client or will be the object of a client's erotic attention. As noted above, the dynamics of therapy ensure this occurs. Still, clinicians tend to underestimate the power of attraction and often deny the possibility that this will even happen; they convince themselves that they are somehow immune to arousal and attraction in clinical settings. Of course they have no reason to doubt this since the majority of practicing professionals report their formal university training did not prepare them for sexual arousal in the clinical realm. Pope, Keith-Spiegel, and Tabachnick (1986), as one example, surveyed psychotherapists about experiences of sexual attraction to clients. Responses indicated that half of the respondents did not receive any guidance or training concerning this issue, and only 9% reported that their training or supervision was adequate. Finally, those who have been practicing in the field for an extended period of time believe they are resistant or even immune to sexual attraction and the risk of dual relationships.

Three psychological factors reinforce the common underestimation of risk for engagement in a sexual boundary violation:

1. the fundamental attribution error;
2. splitting; and
3. believing current preventative measures are sufficient and as such nothing else can be done to decrease risk.

The Fundamental Attribution Error

The fundamental attribution error, a concept that came into common parlance by Ross (1977), states that we have a cognitive disposition to overemphasize personal characteristics and ignore situational factors when judging others' behavior. Thus a person's "bad" behavior reflects their true underlying personality; situational factors are disregarded. Professionals and the organizations in which they practice configure transgressing clinicians as "bad apples," mistakenly hired into the field and who need to be removed as quickly as possible. Even more, these boundary violating clinicians are perceived as irredeemable and beyond the efforts of any form of rehabilitation. Circumstances leading to a boundary violation are elided regardless of the fact that situational antecedents always occur. Smart, compassionate, and empathic people do not destroy their lives and that of involved patients without specific situational factors insidiously motivating behavior. Through use of the fundamental attribution error however, clinicians can rest easy believing they would *never* engage in the same behavior and that there must be something seriously wrong with those individuals allowing it to occur. These former clinicians underestimate the influence and outright power of situational factors and discount the possibility that they too could be swept up into a boundary violation.

Splitting

The second reason clinicians ignore risk builds upon the fundamental attribution error, and this is the well-known defense mechanism of splitting, which allows us to divide people or beliefs into good or bad and positive or negative. Upon learning that a current or past colleague, a trusted professor, or a well-respected leader in the field has engaged in a sexual boundary violation, the mind, unable to tolerate uncertainty and hold opposing ideas (i.e., a person I trust and admire engaged in unethical and injurious behavior), over-comes the complexity by simply allowing us to focus on only the bad aspects of the transgressor. We immediately and harshly judge clinicians engaging in sexual boundary violations as evil, nefarious, incompetent, damaged, and/or sick. While it would be comforting to conclude that offending professionals have severe characterological problems, the research is very clear and finds a far more worrisome conclusion: risk is based on an ever-changing conflux of clinician characteristics, client characteristics, the nature of the therapeutic relationship in general, an agency's milieu, supervisory relations, even uncon-scious factors. Still, professionals of all disciplines minimize or outright deny this risk. It is so much easier for the human brain to simply ignore all of these factors, deride the transgressing clinician, and move on with hubris that "I" would never engage in similar behavior. We see here a split into the ubiq-uitous "us and them" with "us" as the good clinicians and "them" as trans-gressors; splitting allows clinicians to ignore their idiosyncratic risk since they do not perceive themselves as being in the same category as transgressing professionals.

Believing Current Preventative Measures Are Sufficient

Clinicians believe current preventative measures are successful or at least can-not be improved upon. Mental health treatment facilities, licensing boards, and professional associations have done what they can to prevent sexual boundary violations. During their university training, prospective mental health professionals learn that sexual boundary violations are never justifi-able. They later sign ethical statements reiterating this directive as part of their licensure process as well as when voluntarily joining professional asso-ciations. Annual or bi-annual ethics trainings, a mandatory requirement for professionals to maintain licensure, continue to stress the edict prohibiting dual relationships. Professionals understand their behavioral restrictions and partake of existing preventative measures; what more, they think, can I do?

The Six Pillars of Prevention

How do we navigate the inherent risks of therapy, our complacency, and a tendency towards self-deception? We will make little progress until we out-right acknowledge four conclusions about sexual violations occurring in the mental health treatment field.

First, *it is difficult to eradicate behavior that is purposefully secreted.* The antecedents leading to a sexual boundary violation as well as the violation itself take place within the parameters of private therapy sessions, in which knowledge and oversight of what is actually occurring behind closed doors is minimal to non-existent for outsiders. According to Gabbard (1996),

> "Among the many ironies of the practice of psychotherapy is that the privacy of the confidential therapist-patient relationship is both the cornerstone of practice and a major risk factor in the development of boundary violations. What transpires in psychotherapy is not observed by anyone other than the two participants."
>
> (p. 316)

Furthermore, a violating clinician frequently manipulates the client into moving their clandestine relationship into other domains to avoid detection; this stealthy maneuvering is very similar to the precautionary measures used to hide an extramarital affair.

Second, *sexual boundary violations continue to occur because of shared silence by all involved parties and witnesses.* Offending clinicians and their client victims are unlikely to self-disclose a sexual boundary violation. The transgressing clinician is of course fearful of consequences, and clients often report they have fallen in love and do not want to hurt their new lover who was in the not too distant past their mental health professional. Other clients are so confused by the experience that they simply do not know how to respond. Those experiencing power differentials between themselves and a clinician, such as those with a large age gap, those with intellectual disabilities, and those mandated to treatment by the legal system, may be too frightened to complain. Even colleagues, whose attention may have been piqued by odd, atypical, or suspicious behaviors of a peer, remain silent. Celenza (2007) determined three primary reasons lead to peer silence: fear of retaliation; confusion as to how to respond; and the desire not to hurt a colleague. Colleagues express uncertainty as to their interpretations of a questionable behavior, state they do not want to become embroiled in a possible lawsuit or investigation, and verbalize unease with being the person to trigger an investigation that could lead to the personal and professional destruction of a friend and colleague.

Third, as described in the introduction, *knowledge of ethical guidelines, licensing directives, and workplace rules does not necessarily stop sexual boundary violations; similarly fear of consequences is a not sufficient deterrent.*

Fourth, and the one likely to cause the most consternation amongst professionals, is acknowledgement that we are all at risk, and this risk is dynamic and constantly changing. *No professional is one hundred percent safe from acting on sexual and romantic attraction occurring in clinical settings.* All of the transgressing clinicians I have worked with state in one form or the other, "I can't believe this happened to me" or "I never thought this would happen to me."

With these four qualifications in mind, what can the field do to reduce sexual boundary violations? Research directs us to six primary pillars for prevention, all of which will be addressed in this text (see Figure 1.2). First, and the most powerful, is clinical *self-refection and self-monitoring.* Clinicians must acknowledge the erotic risks inherent in therapy, learn to accept that their risk for engagement in boundary violations is not an unchanging state, and understand that a sexual boundary violation is the end result of a complex process. Risk is dynamic and constantly in flux; those at low risk today might be at much higher risk several months in the future. Also, sexual boundary violations do not simply happen but are instead preceded by a series of fantasies, distorted thoughts, and escalating boundary crossings. Clinicians, upon recognizing attraction to a patient, should seek supervision and consultation quickly. This sounds easy, but in actual practice it is far more difficult than one would imagine; according to aforementioned Gabbard (1996), "[I]nternal monitoring [is] a form of scrutiny that will always be imperfect and will always be subject to the vagaries of countertransference, bias, denial, and unconscious wishes for the patient to meet the therapist's needs" (p. 316).

Since self-refection and self-monitoring are frequently foiled by self-deception, this leads to the second pillar of prevention: *education and training.* Most training on sexual boundary violations consists of reminders that the behavior is unethical, harmful, and increasingly illegal; it is the rare clinician who does not know this already. However, the majority of clinicians never receive comprehensive education on the topic in their college/university trainings, workplace-specific trainings, and continuing education requirements. This book thus offers guidance as to:

• risk assessment for poor sexual decision-making;
• a protocol for engaging in better sexual decision-making. Erotic boundary violations are the end result of a process subsuming thoughts, emotions, and physical sensations in which step by step a clinician gradually and imperceptibly progresses towards this outcome;
• use of self-talk to exit sexual situations;
• management of sexual arousal;
• discovering how sexual activity is often used as a substitution for other unfulfilled basic needs; and
• using attraction and arousal for personal and professional growth.

Enhanced supervision and/or consultation is the next pillar of prevention. Competent supervision increases the likelihood that supervisees will disclose erotic attraction to clients, but this requires supervisors who are both knowledgeable and comfortable with the topic. Without supervision, clinicians will flounder in confused silence about attraction to clients. Clinicians can seek supervision and consultation at any point, but embarrassment and shame, lack of knowledge as how to manage arousal in clinical work, and overestimation of one's ability to manage it lead them to remain silent. Clinicians must learn how to utilize supervision to address topics they would rather not, including arousal and attraction to a client. According to Gabbard (1996),

> All therapists should also be trained in valuing the supervisory or consultation process and knowing when to use it. One precept that should be ingrained in all therapists is that anything they are doing with, or saying to, a patient should be something that they could feel comfortable sharing with a supervisor. If something is going on that they feel cannot be shared, this is a warning signal that must be taken seriously.
>
> (pp. 319–20)

Still, successful supervision is not the sole onus of clinicians, and supervisors too must actively create a relationship safe for disclosure. A clinician, aware that they have entered a slippery slope of attraction and arousal, may desire supervisory input, but a paucity of supervisors both trained and comfortable with the topic is a recurrent and serious impediment. A clinician will not discuss attraction to a client with a supervisor with whom they feel unsafe. Conversely, Paxton, Lovett, and Riggs (2001), in their surveys of practicing psychotherapists, determined those who had past supervisors willing to discuss sexual attraction in therapy reported they were better prepared for these occurrences.

The fourth pillar is the *creation of organizations resistant to violations*. All organizations are replete with practices that deter or promote progress towards sexual boundary violations, including formal policy and its implementation, modeling by co-workers and supervisors, and the general culture of a workplace. Just as workplaces that implicitly communicate tolerance of sexual harassment experience higher levels of this behavior, organizations that tolerate less serious boundary crossings (e.g., socially texting clients after working hours) make it seem less worrisome to clinicians when they themselves engage in the same behavior. Boundary crossings almost always precede a sexual boundary violation. Furthermore, inconsistent or reactive organizational handling of clinician arousal leads to lack of disclosure. A clinician is unlikely to expose themself as having attraction to a client if aware the immediate and axiomatic response will be to place the patient – the one they care about – with a new mental health worker and/or disciplinary action. Colleagues and other clients too are unlikely to disclose concerns if they know the involved mental health practitioner is likely to lose a license, their job, and career, and that there is no second chance or option of rehabilitation. In sum, at a meta-level of analysis the culture of an organization affects counterproductive behavior occurring within it (Boye and Jones, 1997), and this text assists readers in understanding organizational factors that facilitate poor sexual decision-making. Context influences sexual decision-making; even our most cherished personal morals and scruples can be elided depending on the circumstances in which we find ourselves.

The fifth pillar is the existence of *professional consequences* for boundary violations. As noted earlier, consequences by themselves do not necessarily sway behavior, particularly behavior that can be successfully hidden. However, they remain one component of a comprehensive prevention plan.

Finally, the sixth pillar is *removal from the field or rehabilitation*, which will be one of the most controversial topics in this book. Predatory clinicians must be removed from the field so as not to amass more victims, but many nonpredatory types are indeed capable of rehabilitation and can return to the workplace with specific restrictions in place.

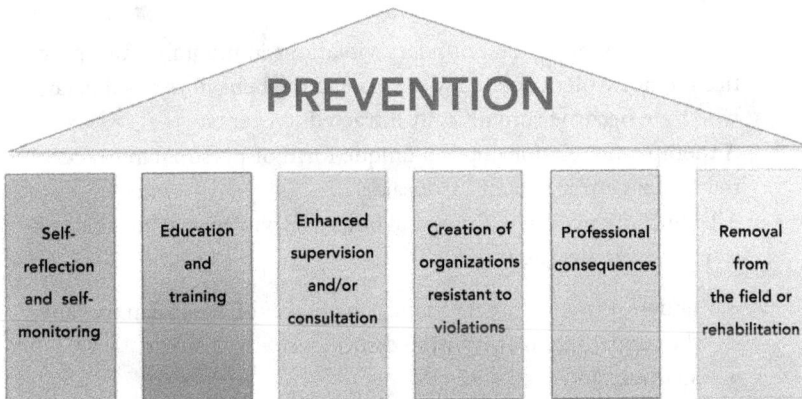

PREVENTION

| Self-reflection and self-monitoring | Education and training | Enhanced supervision and/or consultation | Creation of organizations resistant to violations | Professional consequences | Removal from the field or rehabilitation |

Figure 1.2 The Six Pillars of Prevention

Reducing sexual boundary violations requires feeling safe in disclosing arousal and attraction *before* it escalates to serious behaviors. All parties, including clinicians, colleagues, supervisors, workplaces, licensing boards, and professional associations have their role to play.

Conclusions

Every clinician is at risk for a boundary violation and the risk potential is dynamic and never permanently fixed. A clinician at low risk today may be at much higher risk several months in the future. The process of therapy fosters intimacy, attraction, and arousal. Risk potential for engaging in a boundary violation is further compounded by underestimation of the frequency and influence of arousal in therapy, the fundamental attribution error, splitting, and a common misperception that current preventative measures are successful or at least cannot be improved upon.

Sexual boundary violations were and continue to be a major problem in the field, and unless changes are implemented we should expect them to be a part the future of mental health treatment. Awareness of consequences, careful self-monitoring, education and training, safe and reliable supervision, organizational integrity, and rehabilitation or removal from the field are the essential components we must incorporate to nullify this prediction.

Summary

- The majority of sexual boundary violations in mental health practice are not violent acts; they are instead the behaviors of clinicians who have become romantically attracted to clients.
- A therapeutic relationship is a unique form of personal interaction that fosters attraction and arousal.
- All clinicians are at risk for sexual boundary violations, but this risk is underestimated due to:

  ○ underestimating the frequency and power of arousal in therapy;
  ○ the fundamental attribution error;
  ○ splitting; and
  ○ believing that current preventative measures cannot be improved upon.

- The only reliable method of reducing sexual boundary violations is to end shared silence. Still, all major parties have understandable, though ultimately counterproductive, reasons for remaining silent.
- There are six pillars of prevention for sexual boundary violations: self-reflection and self-monitoring; education and training; supervision and/or consultation; creation of organizations resistant to violations; professional consequences; and removal from the field or rehabilitation for violating professionals.

References

Boye, M.W., & Jones, J. W. (1997). Organizational culture and employee counterproductivity. In R.A. Giacalone & J. Greenberg (Eds.), *Antisocial behaviors in organizations* (pp. 172–184). Thousand Oaks, California: Sage.

Celenza, A. (2007). *Sexual boundary violations.* Lanham, Maryland: Jason Aronson.

Gabbard, G. O. (1996). Lessons to be learned from the study of sexual boundary violations. *American Journal of Psychotherapy, 50*(3), 311–322.

Honig, R. G., & Barron, J. W. (2013). Restoring institutional integrity in the wake of sexual boundary violations: A case study. *Journal of the American Psychoanalytic Association, 61*(5), 897–924.

Paxton, C., Lovett, J., & Riggs, M. L. (2001). The nature of professional training and perceptions of adequacy in dealing with sexual feelings in psychotherapy: Experiences of clinical faculty. *Ethics & Behavior, 11*(2), 175–189.

Pope, K. S., Keith-Spiegel, P., & Tabachnick, B. G. (1986). Sexual attraction to clients: The human therapist and the (sometimes) inhuman training system. *American Psychologist, 41*(2), 147–158.

Ross, L. (1977). The intuitive psychologist and his shortcomings: Distortions in the attribution process. In L. Berkowitz Ed., *Advances in experimental social psychology* (Vol 10, pp. 173–220). New York: Academic Press.

Schwartz, R. S., & Olds, J. (2002). A phenomenology of closeness and its application to sexual boundary violations: A framework for therapists in training. *American Journal of Psychotherapy, 56*(4), 480–493.

Simon, R. I. (1989). Sexual exploitation of patients: How it begins before it happens. *Psychiatric Annals, 19*(2), 104–112.

The Boundary Violation Cycle

2

The history of psychological research on sexual deviance is replete with the creation of typologies – classification systems of offenders. For example, recognized typologies of child sexual abusers include pedophilic and nonpedophilic. Rapist typologies include relationships to victims (stranger or acquaintance) and impulsive versus planned offenders. More recently typologies of female and internet offenders were developed. It is then not too surprising that early work on clinicians engaging in sexual boundary violations began by identifying typologies of transgressors.

An early typology developed by Schoener and Gonsiorek (1988) listed six categories of sexually transgressing therapists:

- **Uninformed/Naïve** – In this group are individuals who lack both knowledge about standards and ethical requirements in their respective fields, and an understanding of the importance of professional boundaries. According to the authors, "ignorance rather than impulsiveness" lead them to a boundary violation (p. 228).
- **Healthy or Mildly Neurotic** – Professionals in this group are responding to situational and proximal stressors, are aware of the unethical nature of their conduct, and are remorseful.
- **Severely Neurotic** – This category contains professionals who use their work to avoid personal longstanding mental health issues, such as depression, anxiety, and/or low self-valuation. These practitioners become over-involved in the lives of their patients, and, for specific clients, situational factors precipitate this enmeshment into sexual dynamics.
- **Impulsive Character Disorder** – Professionals with significant histories of impulse control problems typify this category; a sexual boundary violation is merely one of many impulsive behaviors characterizing their lives.

- **Sociopathic or Narcissistic** – These individuals present with significant histories of exploiting others for their own gratification. They act deliberately, are experts in manipulation, and know how to obfuscate their unethical and antisocial behaviors.
- **Psychotic or Borderline Personality Disorder** – These professionals have poor social judgment and reality testing and typically have long histories of unpredictable behavior.

Assalian (2003) too developed a typology capturing the motives and behaviors of transgressing professionals:

- **Incidental offenders** – Those who impulsively behave in a sexually inappropriate manner and for which there is only one known occurrence of the behavior.
- **Interpersonal offenders** – Professionals motivated to establish a close, intimate, and long-lasting relationship, and who purposefully attempt to minimize exploitation or abuse. These are typically professionals who fall in love with a client.
- **Narcissistic offenders** – These individuals' behavior evince strong needs for attachment, admiration, approval, validation, love, and attention.
- **Compensatory offenders** – Professionals who engage in boundary transgressions to fulfill unmet needs for physical closeness, affection, and sexual relations.
- **Exploitive offenders** – Individuals who use their position of authority and power to fulfill their needs.
- **Angry offenders** – Professional males who target women as a means of acting out strong feelings of hostility, rage, and resentment toward this gender.
- **Sadistic offenders** – Individuals who obtain pleasure by provoking suffering.

Celenza (2007) created a simplified typology consisting of a mere two categories. First, psychopathic predatory transgressors, who engage in sexual activity with numerous clients over the course of their careers and demonstrate little remorse or guilt for their actions. Second, there are one-time offenders, a group the author describes as, "[M]ore like you and me than generally accepted or than is comfortable to acknowledge." (p. 10). This latter category has a high potential for rehabilitation while the former remains a threat and needs to be removed from the field.

While the above typologies are frequently cited in the literature for the direction they offered in the early and then nascent research with transgressing mental health professionals, they are rarely used in treatment other than for guiding decision-making as to risk of reoffending. For example, predatory offenders are recognized as high-risk for reoffending, unlikely to benefit from rehabilitative efforts, and require revocation of their professional licensure. This chapter builds upon these earlier efforts by introducing the Boundary Violation Cycle, a chain of thoughts, feelings, and behaviors that can ultimately lead a clinician to engage in a sexual boundary violation. A cycle also suggests that the pattern is likely to repeat itself. Rather than examine the characteristics of violators it instead examines the *process* leading to the outcome.

Cycles have been used to explain many serious behavioral problems. Walker's (1979) groundbreaking study on domestic violence for example led to the formulation of a battering cycle comprised of three distinct stages. Norris (1989) found a self-perpetuating circular pattern for serial killers, who often rotate through seven stages. O'Farrell and Fals-Stewart (2006) highlighted a destructive cycle in couples struggling with one partner's substance use consisting of four stages.

Sex offender treatment too relies heavily on cycles, often referred to as offense cycles, both as explanatory models in conceptualizing sexual acts and as a clinical tool. Kahn (1990) described a commonly used four-phase cycle. During the first phase, *building up*, individuals fantasize about offending, devise plans as to how to make it occur, and commit to offending. The second phase consists of the *actual sexual assault*. This is followed by *justification*, the third phase, in which the offender experiences guilt, fear of consequences, and promises to never to do it again. Finally, during the *pretend normal* phase, offenders return to a normal routine and act as if the offense never occurred. However, unhealthy arousal and fantasy eventually make an appearance and the cycle repeats.

Similarities of Behavioral Cycles

Behavioral cycles – regardless of the specific behaviors – share several principles. First, they posit that indicated behaviors do not occur without reason. Many mental health professionals engaging in sexual contact with a client report, "It just happened" or "I don't know how this happened." The majority are being honest since they are only partially aware of the interconnected chain of contextual factors, thoughts, feelings, and behaviors that led to progression to a sexual act. Similarly, batterers, serial killers, substance using spouses, and sex offenders often claim there is no comprehendible explanation for their actions, but many indeed follow a specific pattern. In short, mental health professionals engaging in sexual contact with clients or patients are not acting impulsively or blinded by passion; their actions do not occur "out of the blue." Instead, most follow the steps of the Boundary Violation Cycle.

Second, cycles are comprised of phases. Carich, Gray, Rombouts, Stone, & Pithers. (2001) reviewed several existing sexual offense cycles and found three general phases. First, the *pre-assault phase* occurs when a person is struggling with troubling thoughts, emotions, fantasies, stress, and/or efforts at self-control; this person is moving in the direction of an offense. Second, the *assault phase* occurs at that point at which a sexual offense happens. Finally, the *post-assault phase* occurs after an offense; here the perpetrator attempts to minimize repercussion, experiences guilt, shame, and fear, and often promises to refrain from similar behaviors in the future. Cycles in general depict a building-up period, acting-out period, and resolution period, and, as we will soon see, the Boundary Violation Cycle follows these same principles.

Third, cycles have momentums of their own. Consider an analogy of a boulder rolling down a steep hill. The boulder picks up momentum as it travels down the slope, and the more it progresses down the slope the more difficult it is to stop (see Figure 2.1).

The same holds true for the Boundary Violation Cycle: the longer one travels along it the more challenging it is to exit it. Each step along the Boundary Violation Cycle entrenches one deeper in the process and makes it far less likely one will be able to stop its momentum.

Fourth, behavioral cycles predict that unless individuals learn how to exit a cycle, they will likely repeat the pattern. Fortunately, one can exit a cycle at any point through a myriad of cognitive and behavioral interventions. Entering a cycle can and often does lead to regrettable behaviors, but it certainly does not have to be the outcome.

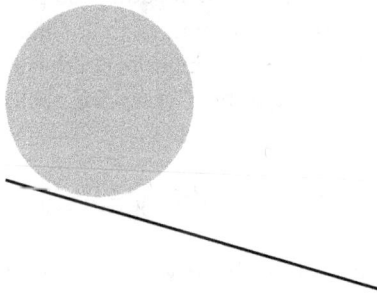

Figure 2.1 The Power of Momentum

The Boundary Violation Cycle

This section will introduce the sexual offense cycle used throughout the book and offers a brief summary of its phases. Later chapters in the text will offer a far more detailed and nuanced description of each phase.

It is only in the past several years that researchers began to investigate the process leading clinicians to engage in sexual boundary violations (e.g., McNulty, Ogden, & Warren, 2013; Tschan, 2013). The Boundary Violation Cycle used throughout this text is based on several models used in offender research and treatment. An original conceptualization by Wolf (1989) has evolved into numerous models. A cycle formulation for child molesters was developed based on offenders' recollections and accounts of their criminal activity (Polaschek & Hudson, 2004). Later research acknowledged that the offense process of those engaging in sexual contact with children was not fully applicable to men who offended against adult victims. This led to the formulation of offense cycles for adult male rapists (Polaschek, Hudson, Ward, & Siegert, 2001). Building upon this earlier work, the offending process of those with intellectual disabilities evolved into clinical enquiry (Courtney, Rose, & Maason, 2006). More recently, it was determined that the offense process for female offenders differs from male rapists as well as offenders against children and new models began to focus on this demographic (Gannon, Rose, & Ward, 2008). Other important contributions to the Boundary Violation Cycle are Finkelhor's (1984) four pre-conditions for offending (motivation to abuse; overcoming internal inhibitions; overcoming external obstacles; and overcoming a victim's resistance) as well as Sullivan's (2002) Spiral of Sexual Abuse, which highlights the key importance of fantasy in offense perpetration.

The Boundary Violation Cycle is a pathway for mental health professionals who know that sexual and romantic relationships with clients are harmful. It does not apply to professionals lacking knowledge that boundary crossings are prohibited nor does it apply to sociopathic and predatory clinicians who purposefully seek out numerous victims in their clinical work, a population that sadly exists and will be described in more depth later in the text. In short, the cycle is pertinent to the majority of practicing clinicians (see Figure 2.2).

Phase One: Risk and Vulnerability Factors Phase

Each individual's idiosyncratic history fosters specific risks, vulnerabilities, and strengths that respectively increase or lower the likelihood of a clinical sexual boundary violation. These include distal developmental

Phase seven: post-violation considerations

Phase one: risk and vulnerability factors

Phase six: sexual boundary violation

Phase two: trigger

Phase five: non-sexual boundary crossings

Phase three: fantasy

Phase four: choosing

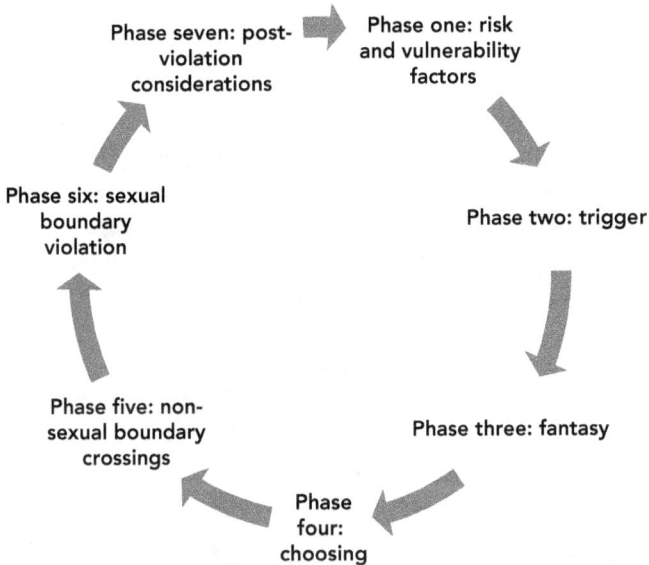

Figure 2.2 The Boundary Violation Cycle

factors such as childhood, adolescent, and early adult sexual experiences and behaviors, contextual environmental factors such as parental modeling and peer group involvement, and biological factors such as impulsivity and risk taking proclivity. As an example, the aforementioned work by Gannon et al. (2008) determined female sex offenders experienced poor familial relations, including physical, emotional, and sexual abuse as part of their upbringing.

In addition to distal risk and vulnerability factors, we must also consider one's more recent and proximal history, which typically ranges from 1 year prior to a boundary violation to moments before its occurrence. This entails recent stressors and significant life events such as relationship issues (e.g., divorce or separation), metal health problems, stress, isolation, loneliness, and general life dissatisfaction. The majority of actuarial findings regarding sexual boundary crossings indicate proximal factors such as current life stress and isolation from colleagues (e.g., working in private practice) are central to their occurrence (Celenza, 2007).

Though every clinician is at risk for a sexual boundary crossing, some are more vulnerable than others. Each clinician brings into their work a history of static and unchanging developmental risk factors as well as current and ongoing dynamic risk influences. Each person's history – both proximal and distal – affects later sexual decision-making and sexual behaviors.

Phase Two: Trigger

Every clinician will work with clients that they find attractive, sexual arousing, and/or romantically stimulating. This is normal, normative, and quite frankly, human. A trigger in the Boundary Violation Cycle is a client who evokes this arousal, and this can be based on appearance, personality, interaction style, or even similarity to figures in one's past. Ladany et al. (1997) interviewed predoctoral psychology interns about their experiences of sexual attraction to clients. Five markers of attraction were found:

- client was physically attractive to them;
- client was a good therapy client (e.g., articulate; introspective);
- client was flirtatious or provocative;
- client was needy or vulnerable and
- client had an attractive personality.

These results are very similar to the earlier findings of Pope, Keith-Spiegel, and Tabachnick (1986), who surveyed practicing psychotherapists about sexual attraction to clients. 87% reported they had been attracted to clients, and characteristics to which they were drawn included (in descending order) physical attractiveness; positive mental/cognitive abilities (e.g., intelligence, creativity); sexual aspects of the client (e.g., sexual histories or sexual material they discussed in therapy); vulnerability, and personality characteristics.

Attraction may occur immediately or develop slowly through working together. In the Ladany et al. (1997) study of predoctoral students, participants reported attraction at first sight was rare and that it typically emerged as treatment progressed.

Phase Three: Fantasy

Sexual fantasy is the most common human sexual experience. There is no doubt that sexual fantasies – whether they are momentary, episodic, violent and aggressive, or tender and loving – can and do influence behavior, a topic that is explored in Chapter 4. For example, fantasies do not lead to a catharsis of libido but instead intensify it. Additionally, fantasy is used to mentally rehearse a desired boundary violation.

A sexual behavior one later regrets almost always begins with fantasy, whether it be fleeting or extending through days, weeks, or months. For many clinicians, sexual and/or romantic fantasies of a particular client become a recurrent, persistent, and distracting presence in their lives. Some may freely engage in fantasies of the client, often including masturbation, while others resist these involvements. Fantasizing is the gateway to poor sexual decision-making and leads to the next phase of the cycle.

Phase Four: Choosing

In this phase of the Boundary Violation Cycle, professionals, recognizing arousal and attraction to a client, either make efforts to avoid progressing along the cycle or engage in faulty and distorted self-talk facilitating advancement towards a violation. Distorted thinking allows them to overcome doubts, fear of consequences, and knowledge that sexual boundary violations are anathema to their field and harmful to clients. Chapter 5 will describe a full list of these distortions and their impact on sexual decision-making. But, for now, to illustrate their influence, consider "fortune telling" also referred to as "predicting the future." Using this specific distortion, clinicians convince themselves that they will not get caught if a boundary violation occurs. Specific examples of fortune telling include:

- "She (the patient) would never tell anybody about this; this will remain between the two of us."
- "Even if this is found out I'll be able to talk my way out of it. Nobody would believe her over me."

The choosing phase of the cycle is the bridge between arousal and fantasy to outright behavior.

Phase Five: Non-Sexual Boundary Crossings

There is significant evidence that non-sexual boundary crossings consistently precede a sexual relationship between a client and mental health professional. Boundary crossings are deviations from standard clinical practice, and two of the most common cited in the literature as preceding a sexual incident are increasing self-disclosure by a professional and social contact between this person and a client outside the confines of therapy (e.g., texting, e-mailing, and phone contact to discuss social and non-clinical matters; meeting for drinks or a meal; and socializing together). Nachmani and Somer (2007) interviewed female patients who had had sexual relationships with their therapists.

They found a slow progression of three boundary crossings: changes in the therapeutic setting (duration of sessions and changes in seating arrangements); self-disclosure by the professional; and alterations in the therapist's attitudes towards the client, including compliments on their personality and appearance.

While a mental health worker may offer money for sex or proposition a client in some other fashion soon after initiating clinical work, this is the behavior of impulsive, antisocial, and/or predatory individuals working with highly vulnerable populations. Even the most alluring, seductive, or sexually solicitous client (or "trigger" using the terminology of the Boundary Violation Cycle) does not lead to physically intimate activity after one or two sessions for the overwhelming majority of professionals even though they may experience arousal, fantasy, and permissive self-talk during this time frame. Mental health professionals know the risks inherent in boundary violations for themselves and their clients. They instead test the possibility of expanding a relationship with a client by subtle and escalating forms of intimacy in both verbal and behavioral forms.

Phase Six: Sexual Boundary Violation

At this phase a singular sexual behavior occurs or a romantic and/or sexual relationship begins. Many immediately think that a sexual boundary violation consists of penis and vagina contact but this requirement is delimiting; such a conceptualization elides the reality of same-sex contact between provider and client or even hands-off behaviors such as masturbating in front of a client. There are instead a myriad of sexual boundary violations and Tschan (2013), as one example, describes three categories of sexual behavior:

- (attempted) penetration (vaginal, anal, oral), genital stimulation; whether with or without ejaculation or orgasm (hands-on);
- sexual impropriety, such as kissing, fondling, taking pictures of intimate body parts, including voyeuristic or exhibitionistic behavior, and presenting pornographic material (hands-off); and
- dating or attempted dating.

A definition by Halter, Brown, and Stone (2007) also offers guidance: "Sexual boundary violations occur wherever a clinical or therapeutic relationship is turned into a sexual or sexualised encounter" (p. 11).

Phase Seven: Post-Violation Considerations

Some clinicians may regret a sexual encounter with a client, possibly as soon as it concludes, while others will appraise it with a positive valuation. Regardless, clinicians now find themselves in an untenable situation, and four processes occur. First, there is an effort at crisis management, including minimizing the possibility of disclosure of the incident to anybody else but the two individuals involved. Many clinicians alert a client to whom they are attracted to the dangers of their romantic and sexual involvement, and they both strategize as to how to work together to protect career and reputation.

Second, clinicians again use distorted thinking to justify and rationalize their behavior. Examples of such self-talk include, "She enjoyed this and wasn't hurt by this;" "We really love each other;" and "Any person in the same situation would do the same thing." Minimization of the negative impact and justification for one's actions are the primary cognitive distortions seen in this phase (Williams, 2005).

Third, clinicians attempt to present to colleagues, supervisors, other patients, and family as if nothing has changed and that no significant event has occurred; life goes on as normal. The sexual offender treatment field calls this a "pretend normal" lifestyle. Finally, transgressing clinicians begin to consider the long-term significance of their boundary violation, particularly if it develops into a romantic relationship. They ask if they can continue working with a client, what this means for an existing relationship with others in their lives (such as a marriage), and whether they can continue in their career.

Exiting the Cycle

The Boundary Violation Cycle offers clinicians an explanatory process model for sexual boundary violations. Similar cycles have been used in offender treatment for decades and they have been found to be clinically valuable for two reasons. First, these models posit that a sexual transgression does not just occur; there are multiple steps leading to this outcome. Knowing that an underlying process of intertwined thought, feelings, and behaviors is occurring allows one to take control of decision-making. One is not simply at the mercy of seemingly chaotic forces leading inexorably to a consequential outcome. Second, and of greater importance, once one recognizes that an underlying process is occurring, a person can map where they are in the cycle and implement a series of corrective measures to change course; at each pre-violation phase of the cycle, whether it be fantasy, choosing, or non-sexual boundary crossings, there exist interventions that can halt progress towards a boundary violation. These are explored throughout the text.

Challenges to the Cycle Model

The Boundary Violation Cycle is one way of conceptualizing sexual attraction and sexual boundary crossings in therapy. It is an imperfect model, and other approaches exist. Typologies of transgressors are one example. A recognized problem with all existing process models, whether they describe rapists, child offenders, female sex offenders, or transgressing mental health professionals, is they are based on post-offense accounts. Transgressors and victims recollect the events leading to a boundary violation or crime, and researchers retrospectively configure recurrent patterns. In short, process models are based on those who have already offended. There is little existing information on the strategies of those who successfully navigate sexual and romantic attraction, but fortunately there are efforts to improve upon this deficit. For example, Martin, Godfrey, Meekums, and Madill (2011) and Luca and Boyden (2014) formulated distinct processes by which clinicians therapeutically and proactively manage sexual attraction in therapy; these will be explored in Chapter 5.

Another challenge to the model is the majority of transgressing clinicians engage in a sexual boundary violation once, and, as such, a linear model would better illustrate the decision-making process. A counterargument is that the once a professional engages romantically and/or sexually with a client this event now becomes part of their sexual history, which is recognized in phase one: risk and vulnerability factors. While the outcome might dissuade some clinicians from acting on arousal in the future, for others the knowledge that they were able to evade consequences might be an additional incentive when convincing themselves to act on their arousal the next time it occurs. Additionally, clinicians who establish romantic relationships with clients that extend through weeks, months, or years continue to recycle through the model as a means of justifying their continued involvement.

Finally, for the purpose of reification, the Boundary Violation Cycle presents phases as if they were discrete occurrences moving in one unalterable direction only. In reality, a clinician may vacillate between one stage and another, moving forward or backward dependent on the changing circumstances. For example, a client's rebuff to a subtle seductive disclosure may lead the clinician back to the fantasy stage. Progression through the cycle is fluid and is certainly not inviolate. The length of time one remains in a particular phase is similarly fluid; a professional may remain in a particular phase for an extended period of time while another lasts for moments. Also, phases are not isolated; progression through the cycle requires continued use of earlier elements. For example, fantasizing does not occur only in the fantasy phase but continues to occur in later phases; even during the choosing and non-sexual boundary crossings phases a person will have fantasies of the intended target. Movement along the cycle is propelled by a complex merging of arousal, fantasy, and distorted thinking, and some of these aspects will predominate over others throughout the cycle.

Conclusions

The majority of information on professional boundary crossings is prescriptive; it exhorts readers to refrain from this activity and lists the myriad of complications that can arise. The Boundary Violation Cycle, in contrast, is one way of examining *the process* that facilitates progress towards boundary transgressions in clinical practice. It is a chain of internal and external events consisting of sexual arousal, fantasies, cognitive distortions, and contextual factors. The process can occur rapidly or extend through months, and, in some cases, years. Still, the further one progresses along the cycle the more difficult it is to extricate oneself from it. Nonetheless, mental health professionals can learn to recognize that they have entered a cycle and take proactive steps to forestall further progression.

Summary

- Much of the history of research into transgressing professionals focused on the development of typologies.
- More recent models attempt to elucidate the process underlying sexual boundary violations.
- Cycles have been used to explain many serious behavioral problems.
- Behavioral cycles share several principles:
  - an indicated behavior does not occur without reason – there is an underlying though likely unrecognized pattern;
  - cycles are comprised of phases;

- o cycles have momentum; and
- o a person can recognize they are on a cycle and exit it.

- The Boundary Violation Cycle is a process model explaining sexual and romantic involvement between mental health professionals and their clients/patients.
- The Boundary Violation Cycle is composed of seven phases:

  - o risk and vulnerability factors;
  - o trigger;
  - o fantasy;
  - o choosing;
  - o non-sexual boundary crossings;
  - o sexual boundary violation; and
  - o post-violation considerations

References

Assalian, P. (2003). Management of professional sexual misconduct: Evaluation and recommendations. *Journal of Sexual & Reproductive Medicine, 3*(3), 89–92.

Carich, M.S., Gray, A., Rombouts, S., Stone, M. & Pithers, W.D. (2001). Relapse prevention and the sexual assault cycle. In M.S. Carich & S.E. Mussack (Eds.), *Handbook for sexual abuser assessment and treatment* (pp. 77–103). Brandon, Vermont: Safer Society Press.

Celenza, A. (2007). *Sexual boundary violations.* Lanham, Maryland: Jason Aronson.

Courtney, J., Rose, J., & Mason, O. (2006). The offence process of sex offenders with intellectual disabilities: A qualitative study. *Sexual Abuse, 18*(2), 169–191.

Finkelhor, D. (1984). *Child sexual abuse: New theory and research.* New York: Free Press, 1984.

Gannon, T. A., Rose, M. R., & Ward, T. (2008). A descriptive model of the offense process for female sexual offenders. *Sexual Abuse, 20*(3), 352–374.

Halter, M., Brown, H., & Stone, J. (2007). Sexual boundary violations by health professionals–An overview of the published empirical literature. Council for Healthcare Regulatory Excellence.

Kahn, T. J. (1990). *Pathways: A guided workbook for youth beginning treatment.* Orwell, VT: Safer Society Press.

Ladany, N., O'Brien, K. M., Hill, C. E., Melincoff, D. S., Knox, S., & Petersen, D. A. (1997). Sexual attraction toward clients, use of supervision, and prior training: A qualitative study of predoctoral psychology interns. *Journal of Counseling Psychology, 44*(4), 413.

Luca, M., & Boyden, M. (2014). An elephant in the room: A grounded theory of experienced psychotherapists' reactions and attitudes to sexual attraction. In M. Luca (Ed.), *Sexual attraction in therapy: Clinical perspectives on moving beyond the taboo* (pp. 193–208). West Sussex, United Kingdom: John Wiley & Sons.

Martin, C., Godfrey, M., Meekums, B., & Madill, A. (2011). Managing boundaries under pressure: A qualitative study of therapists' experiences of sexual attraction in therapy. *Counselling and Psychotherapy Research*, *11*(4), 248–256.

McNulty, N., Ogden, J., & Warren, F. (2013). 'Neutralizing the patient': Therapists' accounts of sexual boundary violations. *Clinical Psychology & Psychotherapy*, *20*(3), 189–198.

Nachmani, I., & Somer, E. (2007). Women sexually victimized in psychotherapy speak out: The dynamics and outcome of therapist-client sex. *Women & Therapy*, *30*(1–2), 1–17.

Norris, J. (1989). *Serial killers*. New York: Anchor Books.

O'Farrell, T.J., & Fals-Stewart, W. (2006). *Behavioral couples therapy for alcoholism and drug abuse*. New York: Guilford.

Polaschek, D. L., & Hudson, S. M. (2004). Pathways to rape: Preliminary examination of patterns in the offence processes of rapists and their rehabilitation implications. *Journal of Sexual Aggression*, *10*(1), 7–20.

Polaschek, D. L., Hudson, S. M., Ward, T., & Siegert, R. J. (2001). Rapists' offense processes: A preliminary descriptive model. *Journal of Interpersonal Violence*, *16*(6), 523–544.

Pope, K. S., Keith-Spiegel, P., & Tabachnick, B. G. (1986). Sexual attraction to clients: The human therapist and the (sometimes) inhuman training system. *American Psychologist*, *41*(2), 147.

Schoener, G. R., & Gonsiorek, J. (1988). Assessment and development of rehabilitation plans for counselors who have sexually exploited their clients. *Journal of Counseling & Development*, *67*(4), 227–232.

Sullivan J. (2002). The spiral of sexual abuse: A conceptual framework for understanding and illustrating the evolution of sexually abusive behavior. *NOTA News*, *41*, 17–21.

Tschan, W. (2013). *Professional sexual misconduct in institutions: Causes and consequences, prevention and intervention*. Boston: Hogrefe Publishing.

Walker, L. E. (1979). *The battered woman*. New York: Harper & Row.

Williams, D. J. (2005). Functions of leisure and recreational activities within a sexual assault cycle: A case study. *Sexual Addiction & Compulsivity*, *12*(4), 295–309.

Wolf, S. C. (1989). A model of sexual aggression/addiction. *Journal of Social Work & Human Sexuality*, *7*(1), 131–148.

Risk and Vulnerability Factors   **3**

The first phase of the Boundary Violation Cycle examines idiosyncratic risks and vulnerabilities for sexual and romantic involvement with a patient. Research on risk is predicated on two general conclusions. First, risk potential consists of a conflux of static and unchanging factors as well as dynamic and malleable factors. For example, Macapagal, Janssen, Fridberg, Finn, and Heiman (2011) conclude there are cognitive, motivational, and personality factors influencing decision-making for high-risk sexual behaviors while Hertlein, Emmers-Sommer, and Kennedy (2014) state individual and socio-demographic factors (e.g., age, education, personality), awareness and likelihood of sanctions, relationship status, and cultural factors are pivotal.

The second conclusion regarding risk factors is that the more that are present the higher the potential for engaging in consequential sexual behavior. Risk assessments for sex offenders, as an example, tabulate a total score based on the number of static and dynamic risk factors present. While some assessments give more weight to specific risk factor over others (e.g., a history of more than one victim), the total score indicates the likelihood of reoffending from very-low risk to high risk in a specified period of time (e.g., within the next year).

Research on risk presents with serious limitations. Foremost among these, except in rare instances, is that it tends to treat risk factors as independent variables and rarely examines the interactions between or among them. Second, most of the research examining sexual risk-taking is based on adolescents, adults engaging in substance use, or sexual offenders. Studies of risk factors for adults without serious mental health concerns or legal involvements are rare. Studies of transgressing professionals are even less available.

General Risk Factors Influencing Sexual Outcomes

This section enumerates general factors influencing sexual decision-making that are applicable to all individuals, including personality characteristics, static historical factors, current dynamic factors, and situational features. In short, this section elucidates the numerous factors that complicate sexual decision-making for humans in general; the next section then narrows our focus to those risks associated with sexual violations in the clinical realm.

Personality Factors

Research has examined the personality traits of those engaging in risky sexual behaviors. Hoyle, Fejfar, and Miller (2000) engaged in a comprehensive review of studies of personality and risk-taking and found sensation seeking – those who seek novel and often-intense experiences in spite of risk – and impulsivity predict involvement in sexual risk-taking. Later studies have repeatedly come to the same conclusions (e.g., Donohew et al., 2000; Kahn, Kaplowitz, Goodman, & Emans, 2002).

Other personality traits leading to poor sexual decision-making include propensity for sexual excitement and the inability to inhibit arousal. Janssen, Vorst, Finn, and Bancroft (2002) studied variability in arousal and ability to inhibit it when confronted with the threat of consequences. Their work concluded that individuals engaging in risky sexual behaviors differ from those who do not by their inability to regulate and inhibit sexual arousal. Some individuals are aroused by a far wider range of stimuli, become aroused much more quickly and intensely than others, and have difficulty managing this arousal.

A similar line of research examines compulsive sexual behavior, consisting of excessive sexual thoughts, sexual urges, or sexual activity causing distress or impairment (Mick & Hollander, 2006). Coleman (1992) identified seven subtypes of compulsive sexual behavior:

- compulsive cruising and multiple partners;
- compulsive fixation on an unattainable partner;
- compulsive autoeroticism (masturbation);
- compulsive use of erotica;
- compulsive use of the Internet for sexual purposes;

- compulsive multiple love relationships; and
- compulsive sexuality in a relationship.

Compulsive sexual behaviors are thought to be a method by which some individuals cope with underlying anxiety.

Distal and Proximal Factors

Each person's idiosyncratic history presents with developmental risk factors. One recurrent finding is a correlation between childhood sexual abuse and adult sexual risk-taking, though the reason for this association remains unclear. One proposed explanatory model is the traumagenic dynamics framework in which childhood sexual abuse leads to maladaptive scripts for adult sexual behavior (Finkelhor & Browne, 1985).

Sexual scripts learned early in life (regardless of one's personal history of victimization), acquired through media, peers, and family modelling, have been implicated in the research as affecting risk-taking propensity. O'Hara, Gibbons, Gerrard, Li, and Sargent (2012), as an example, found that exposure to sexual content in films, most of which is portrayed in an unrealistic and/or risk-promoting manner, predicted age of sexual debut and sexual sensation-seeking. Common sexual scripts learned include male domination of females (Malamuth, 1986); beliefs that the sexual urges of men are uncontrollable (Flood & Pease, 2009); gender roles supporting aggressiveness, toughness, fearlessness, and violence as core characteristics of masculinity (Eagly & Steffen, 1986), and male entitlement and rigid gender roles (Heise, 1998).

A more proximal risk factor is substance use. The association between substance use and sexual activity has been long recognized, and some of the common assertions regarding the influence of substance use on sexual behavior include that it (Calsyn, Berns, Hatch-Maillette, & Tross, 2009):

- relaxes/disinhibits, so helps one to approach potential partners;
- disinhibits possible partners to be more open to sexual advances;
- increases sexual desire of partners;
- can make partners willing to have sex for drug use;
- delays orgasm;
- increases sexual desire;
- increases sexual sensation;
- intensifies orgasm;

- disinhibits both partners, so as to be more sexually adventurous; and
- leads to firmer erections.

A 2011 review of research on sex offending and substance use determined that approximately a quarter to half of sex offenders appeared to be intoxicated at the time of the offense (Kraanen & Emmelkamp, 2011). Alcohol, in fact, is more closely linked to sexual violence than any other drug (Califano, 1999). Intoxicating substances also lead to non-aggressive sexual risk-taking. For example, using a sample of heterosexual men engaged in substance abuse treatment, researchers found 73.3% reported they had sex under the influence in the prior 90 days, and 39.1% endorsed sex under the influence during their most recent sexual event. Sex under the influence at the most recent event was more likely to involve anal intercourse, sex with a casual partner, and less condom use (Calsyn et al., 2010).

Acute and chronic stress also affects sexual decision-making. Prolonged exposure to stress not only affects physiological functioning, such as the immune system, but cognitive functioning as well. It appears to disrupt executive functioning, including tasks such as working memory, retrieval of information from memory, and attention. Stress also impairs the ability to consider the costs and benefits of one's choices; decision-making while stressed can be disorganized (LeBlanc, 2009; Preston, Buchanan, Stansfield, & Bechara, 2007; Starcke & Brand, 2012).

Situational Factors

Sexual behaviors do not occur in a vacuum but are instead influenced by situational considerations. For example, the majority of college and university-based sexual assaults occur in private places (e.g., a parked car; fraternity houses) rather than public locations (Söchting, Fairbrother, & Koch, 2004). A rich research base on organizational factors leading to sexual harassment in the workplace similarly evinces the influence of the milieu on sexual decision-making. These will be discussed in depth in Chapter 10 but, for now, the availability and ease of grievance procedures for sexual harassment correlates with frequency of the behavior.

Characteristics of the person to whom one is aroused also influence decision-making. Recall from Chapter 2 that the majority of mental health professionals report attraction to a client based on characteristics such as physical attractiveness and personality characteristics. Related to this, each person has their own set of sexual arousal templates, highly personal sources of sexual arousal including body types, body parts, physical characteristics (e.g., hair or muscularity), specific activities (e.g., cheerleading), objects (e.g., clothing or uniforms), personality characteristics, and even cultural designations (e.g., Asian women) (Carnes, 2001). A person is far more likely to be aroused and desire sexual contact when faced with a person or event that activates his or her erotic templates. Finally, a potential sexual partner's willingness to engage in such a relationship also influences the sexual decision-making process. The more likely this person is to comply, acquiesce, or even seek sexual contact, the more likely a sexual outcome is to actually occur.

Summary of General Risk Factors Influencing Sexual Outcomes

In summary we can see that sexual decision-making is complex and influenced by a myriad of factors. It involves more than logically weighing costs and benefits. Personality traits, idiosyncratic proximal and distal risk factors, and situational influences frequently make it very difficult to modulate arousal and make wise sexual decisions.

Professional Risk Factors Influencing Sexual Outcomes

While there is robust research on general risk factors affecting sexual decision-making, research on risk factors for mental health professionals and boundary violations is relatively sparse. Still, efforts have been made to synthesize available literature (e.g., Norris, Gutheil, & Strasburger (2003); Halter, Brown, & Stone (2007); Celenza (2007)). The most noted risk factors in the literature are:

- **Ignoring and denying one's potential risk** – Denying one's risk is a harbinger of poor sexual decision-making in clinical practice. All professionals are at risk for sexual boundary violations regardless of their education, training, and number of years in the field.
- **Being a heterosexual male mental health professional** – The majority of professional sexual boundary violators are heterosexual males. This finding mirrors sexual aggression and violence in general, in which males are typically perpetrators and females are victims. Women presenting with low self-esteem, a history of difficult relationships with males, and histories of sexual trauma, including sexual abuse, are particularly

vulnerable. Somer and Saadon (1999) interviewed female client victims and found that respondents reported retrospectively perceiving it as a romantic affair. The researchers also determined that, for some, the therapist was their only human bond at the time, and they engaged in "desperate erotic attachments" (p.508) with a clinician. In general, men are more likely than women to agree with myths and beliefs supportive of violence against women, perceive a narrower range of behaviors as violent, blame and show less empathy for the victim, minimize the harms associated with physical and sexual assault, and see behaviors constituting violence against women as less serious, inappropriate, or damaging (Flood & Pease, 2009). This conclusion does not negate the presence of female professional boundary transgressors; they do exist, including predatory females, but the number of male offenders undoubtedly dwarfs them. Giovazolias and Davis (2001) remind us that a focus on males elides female arousal in therapy and places an even greater taboo upon this topic; this leads to more discomfort and shame for female mental health workers experiencing attraction and less likelihood that they will reach out to colleagues and supervisors for guidance.

- **Immediate life circumstances of a clinician** – Other findings regarding professional transgressors are that they are mid-career, isolated in their practices, and have little supervision. Two risk factors particularly highlighted in the literature are:

  o *Life crises* – Life crises can precipitate boundary violations for professionals at all career levels, and these include relationship problems, serious illness either for oneself or a loved one, or loss through death.

  o *Life transitions* – Transitions can be related to work, such as promotion or job loss, or result from events outside the professional domain, such as financial reversals. As an example, early-career practitioners may experience a particular set of stressors including establishing a practice and learning to balance home and work life.

Lamb, Catanzaro, and Moorman (2003) interviewed psychologists who had disclosed past sexual involvement with clients, supervisees, and students. They determined that dissatisfaction with their personal life was a precipitating circumstance preceding these violations. Examples include, "I was depressed and alienated from my marital family"; "I was lonely, recently divorced, wanted to be loved and felt insecure", and "[M]y mother was dying, I was in a new job, had a new baby, and I was vulnerable" (p. 105).

- **Client vulnerability** – In general, the more vulnerable a client or patient, the higher the risk of victimization. Capawana (2016), using a social justice approach, states that those patients with greater power differentials between themselves and therapists – children, youths, those with a vast age difference between the clinician and themselves, those with intellectual disabilities, and those mandated to treatment by the legal system – are more likely to be the recipients of unwanted sexual attention and boundary violations.

- **Lack of training and education** – While there is a consensus that knowing the ethical and legal requirements of one's respective mental health profession does not by itself protect against romantic and sexual involvement with clients, they nonetheless remain part of a comprehensive prevention protocol. Berkman, Turner, Cooper, Polnerow, and Swartz (2000) found that while 87% of the social work students engaged in their study had received education on professional ethics and dual relationships in general, only a small proportion (23%) reported discussing sexual ethics in classroom settings and even less in field placements. These same students often mistakenly claimed that mitigating circumstances allowed for sexual contact, such as that a clinical relationship had ended more than 5 years earlier or when a social worker did not engage in psychotherapy with a client but had only assisted in obtaining concrete services. Most of the students in this study felt unprepared to deal with sexual feelings from or towards a client. Echoing this, Harris and Hays (2008) advised that increasing professionals' comfort with sexual topics is the cornerstone to reducing sexual boundary violations.

- **Lack of supervision** – The overwhelming majority of those in the mental health field do not present issues of attraction in supervision. Similarly, supervisors rarely ask questions about the topic primarily because they are uncomfortable with the topic of erotic attraction, do not have enough information to address the topic, and/or are fearful that bringing up this topic could be misinterpreted by a supervisee as a sexual overture. Regardless, Paxton, Lovett, and Riggs (2001) recommend supervisory modeling of the beliefs that sexual feelings are a normal, expected part of any human relationship and must be anticipated and planned for to help therapists feel prepared for these inevitable circumstances. Based on this conclusion, and many similar to it, there is a call to improve supervision on sexual topics.

Other professional boundary violation risk factors have been noted in the literature, but there is less of a consensus regarding them. These include:

- **Clinician characteristics** – Celenza (2007), a leading researcher on professional boundary violations, postulates that many breaches stem from unconscious intrapsychic conflicts of which the offender is unaware. Her work with transgressing professionals informs us that most were capable and competent throughout their careers; violations occurred at a particular time due to transference/countertransference with a particular client at a stressful time in the clinician's life. Transference and countertransference, the causal factors for boundary violations according to psychodynamic practitioners, are explored in Chapter 6. Celenza also notes a recurrence of longstanding narcissistic vulnerability, unresolved anger toward authority figures, childhood histories of emotional deprivation and sexualized overstimulation, and a family history of boundary transgressions (2007).
- **Specific clinical dynamics** – As discussed in Chapter 1, sexual attraction is part of the human condition and inevitably finds its way into the consulting room. A therapeutic relationship is a unique form of intimacy and as such can foster erotic tension. Some forms of clinical interaction however may be riskier than others. Hoencamp (1990), for example, described the heightened risk of hypnotherapy. Rodgers (2011) differentiated between risks in psychodynamic versus other treatment approaches. Power differentials might also increase risk. Thoreson, Shaughnessy, and Frazier (1995), as an example, determined that male counselors were more likely to engage in sexual relationships when they held high-power roles. Finally, long-term treatment appears to pose more risk than short-term interventions due to extended opportunity for fostering interpersonal intimacy. Recall that Ladany et al. (1997) found attraction at first sight was rare and that it typically emerged as treatment progressed.
- **Ambiguity about what constitutes a professional relationship** – Clients often enter treatment having a limited understanding of what the process entails. Even those with previous therapy experiences may have worked with a professional using a very different approach and therapeutic modality. Additionally, many people base their idea of therapy on media representations, which often present sexual boundary violations as common occurrences. In one study Gharaibeh (2005) examined images in commercially available films and determined therapists were portrayed as mainly male (71.2%), and middle-aged (50.8%), and that 23.7% of them violated sexual boundaries.
- **"Small town issues"** – In the confines of small-town settings, providers and patients will frequently encounter one another in nonprofessional

settings, which can lead to overlapping relationships. Note that "small town issues" are not necessarily delimited to this eponymous descriptor. Those sharing particular subcultures (e.g., LGBT+ individuals) are similarly more likely to encounter one another in out-of-office settings, even when living in more populous areas.

- **Drug and alcohol use** – While some clinicians might arrive at a session in an intoxicated state and place clients at immediate risk, more likely scenarios include use of drugs and alcohol to progress through the sexual boundary violation cycle. A clinician might initiate social contact via texting after several drinks have lowered inhibitions. Similarly, clients and professionals who have already engaged in a less-serious boundary crossing, such as having a meal together, may find planned friendly conversation quickly progressing to more intimate contact after use of an intoxicating substance.

Summary of Professional Risk Factors

Based on a review of available literature, six factors are most predictive of a professional sexual boundary violation: minimizing or outright denying one's risk potential; being a heterosexual male therapist working with female clients; the immediate life circumstances of the practitioner; working with a vulnerable patients; and lack of training and supervision. As for the other factors noted in this chapter (clinician characteristics; specific clinical dynamics; ambiguity about what constitutes a professional relationship; "small town issues"; and drug and alcohol use) we remain uncertain as to their power and influence. Rarely do these risk factors occur in isolation and professionals may experience an unanticipated convergence of many of the above. Figure 3.1 details some self-assessment questions that clinicians could use when determining risk.

Conclusions

There is agreement that sexual boundary violations are a result of a confluence of personality, proximal, distal, and situations factors. Even incidents that seem to happen "in the heat of the moment" are grounded on a myriad of factors of which a clinician is often oblivious to but nonetheless exist; some are obfuscated from one's awareness and others are so obvious and commonplace that clinicians believe they can be dismissed without consideration (e.g.,

Risk Self-Assessment Qustions:

- What are the important stressors in your life, and what steps are you taking to resolve or to cope with them?
- Are you engaged in alcohol or use of intoxicating substances?
- Have you had specific training/education on sexual boundary violations?
- Do you minimize your risk potential for engaging in a sexual boundary violation?
- Do you have a history of using sexual activity to improve your mood and/or reduce anxiety?
- Are you high in sensation seeking and/or impulsivity?
- Do you have a difficult time regulating your sexual arousal?
- Are you working with a client you find arousing, either sexually or romantically?
- Has a client revealed their sexual or romantic interest in you?
- Do you live in a small town or are part of a subculture in which unplanned non-clinical encounters with clients frequently occur or in which dual relationships might arise?
- Does your primary satisfaction come from your work with therapy clients?
- Do you have more clients than required?
- Are you lonely and feeling as if your needs are not being met by anyone?
- Do you have a circle of friends to whom you can turn for support?
- Do you have a circle of friends with whom you engage in pleasurable social activities?
- Do you have one or more close friends in whom you could confide about fears, anxieties, and self-doubts?
- Do you have a trusted supervisor or colleague with whom you could discuss sexual attraction to a client?

Adapted from Hamilton and Spruill (1999)

Figure 3.1 Risk Self-Assessment Questions

a heterosexual male professional working with a female patient). There is also agreement that risk potential fluctuates. While distal and personality factors are fairly fixed, proximal and situational factors can and do change, often quickly and with little time for preparation.

Several limitations are noted in the research. First, we have yet to determine the influence of several significant general risk factors on clinical decision-making. The general risk factors noted in this chapter include personality factors, childhood sexual abuse, substance use, and the impact of stress. As one example, do clinicians presenting with compulsive sexual behaviors or having difficulty inhibiting arousal engage in more boundary violations than those who do not have these concerns? Common sense would indicate an increased likelihood, but there is no evidence to bolster or counter this contention.

A second concern is that studies of female boundary violators are sparse, and at this point we are uncertain if many of the factors listed in this chapter are equally relevant for female clinicians. There will no doubt be an overlap between the genders as to risk factors but there will likely be other as-of-yet unknown factors more applicable to female clinicians.

Finally, while we know the risk factors most predictive of a boundary violation, research tends to look at these as independent variables and rarely in combination. This practice sheds little light as to why most clinicians experiencing these same risk factors in their practices do not transgress boundaries. Future research will thus be moving in the direction of multi-causal explanatory models, particularly immediate situational factors that seem to so heavily sway sexual decision-making.

Summary

- The first phase of the Boundary Violation Cycle examines idiosyncratic risks and vulnerabilities.
- Research on risk factors is predicated on two general conclusions:
  - risk potential consists of a conflux of static and unchanging factors as well as dynamic and malleable factors; and
  - the more risk factors present, the higher the potential for engaging in consequential sexual behavior.

- General risk factors for poor sexual decision-making include:
  - personality factors such as sensation seeking, impulsivity, propensity for sexual excitement, the inability to inhibit arousal, and sexual compulsivity;
  - proximal and distal factors, including childhood sexual abuse, substance use, and chronic and acute stress; and

- situational factors such as organizational milieu and the characteristics of a possible romantic/sexual partner, including their willingness to engage in this behavior.

- The risk factors most noted for professional sexual boundary violations are:
  - ignoring and denying one's potential risk;
  - being a heterosexual male mental health professional with female clients;
  - immediate life circumstances of a clinician, including life crises and transitions;
  - having vulnerable clients;
  - lack of training and education; and
  - lack of supervision.

- Risk factors for boundary violations having less consensus in the research are:
  - clinician characteristics;
  - specific clinical dynamics;
  - ambiguity about what constitutes a professional relationship;
  - "small town issues"; and
  - drug and alcohol use.

- Studies of female boundary violators are sparse, and it is uncertain if many of the factors listed in this chapter are equally relevant for female clinicians.
- Risk potential fluctuates. While distal and personality factors are fairly fixed, proximal and situational factors can and do change.

References

Berkman, C. S., Turner, S. G., Cooper, M., Polnerow, D., & Swartz, M. (2000). Sexual contact with clients: Assessment of social workers' attitudes and educational preparation. *Social Work*, 45(3), 223–235.

Califano, J. A. (1999). *Dangerous liaisons: Substance abuse and sex.* The National Center on Addiction and Substance Abuse at Columbia University (CASA).

Calsyn, D.A., Berns, S.B., Hatch-Maillette, M.A., & Tross, S. (2009). *Real Men Are Safe (REMAS): A gender-focused HIV and sexual risk reduction intervention for men in substance abuse treatment* (Seattle, WA: CTN Pacific Northwest Node, Alcohol & Drug Abuse Institute, University of Washington).

Calsyn, D. A., Cousins, S. J., Hatch-Maillette, M. A., Forcehimes, A., Mandler, R., Doyle, S. R., & Woody, G. (2010). Sex under the influence of drugs or alcohol: Common for men in substance abuse treatment and associated with high-risk sexual behavior. *The American Journal on Addictions, 19*(2), 119–127.

Capawana, M. R. (2016). Intimate attractions and sexual misconduct in the therapeutic relationship: Implications for socially just practice. *Cogent Psychology, 3*(1), 1–13.

Carnes, P. (2001). *Out of the shadows: Understanding sexual addiction.* Center City: Minnesota Hazelden Publishing.

Celenza, A. (2007). *Sexual boundary violations.* Lanham, Maryland: Jason Aronson.

Coleman, E. (1992). Is your patient suffering from compulsive sexual behavior?.*Psychiatric Annals, 22*(6), 320–325.

Donohew, L., Zimmerman, R., Cupp, P. S., Novak, S., Colon, S., & Abell, R. (2000). Sensation seeking, impulsive decision-making, and risky sex: Implications for risk-taking and design of interventions. *Personality and Individual Differences, 28*(6), 1079–1091.

Eagly, A. H., & Steffen, V. J. (1986). Gender and aggressive behavior: A meta-analytic review of the social psychological literature. *Psychological Bulletin, 100*(3), 309.

Finkelhor, D., & Browne, A. (1985). The traumatic impact of child sexual abuse: A conceptualization. *American Journal of Orthopsychiatry, 55*(4), 530–541.

Flood, M., & Pease, B. (2009). Factors influencing attitudes to violence against women. *Trauma, vViolence, & Abuse, 10*(2), 125–142.

Gharaibeh, N. M. (2005). The psychiatrist's image in commercially available American movies. *Acta Psychiatrica Scandinavica, 111*(4), 316–319.

Giovazolias, T., & Davis, P. (2001). How common is sexual attraction towards clients? The experiences of sexual attraction of counselling psychologists toward their clients and its impact on the therapeutic process. *Counselling Psychology Quarterly, 14*(4), 281–286.

Halter, M., Brown, H., & Stone, J. (2007). *Sexual boundary violations by health professionals– An overview of the published empirical literature.* London, United Kingdom: Council for Healthcare Regulatory Excellence.

Harris, S. M., & Hays, K. W. (2008). Family therapist comfort with and willingness to discuss client sexuality. *Journal of Marital and Family Therapy, 34*(2), 239–250.

Heise, L. L. (1998). Violence against women: An integrated, ecological framework. *Violence Against Women, 4*(3), 262–290.

Hertlein, K. M., Emmers-Sommer, T. M., & Kennedy, M. A. (2014). Testing a model predicting risky sexual behavior. *Marriage & Family Review, 50*(2), 107–128.

Hoencamp, E. (1990). Sexual abuse and the abuse of hypnosis in the therapeutic relationship. *International Journal of Clinical & Experimental Hypnosis, 38*(4), 283–297.

Hoyle, R. H., Fejfar, M. C., & Miller, J. D. (2000). Personality and sexual risk taking: A quantitative review. *Journal of Personality, 68*(6), 1203–1231.

Janssen, E., Vorst, H., Finn, P., & Bancroft, J. (2002). The Sexual Inhibition (SIS) and Sexual Excitation (SES) Scales: I. measuring sexual inhibition and excitation proneness in men. *Journal of Sex Research, 39*(2), 114–126.

Kahn, J. A., Kaplowitz, R. A., Goodman, E., & Emans, S. J. (2002). The association between impulsiveness and sexual risk behaviors in adolescent and young adult women. *Journal of Adolescent Health, 30*(4), 229–232.

Kraanen, F. L., & Emmelkamp, P. M. (2011). Substance misuse and substance use disorders in sex offenders: A review. *Clinical Psychology Review, 31*(3), 478–489.

Ladany, N., O'Brien, K. M., Hill, C. E., Melincoff, D. S., Knox, S., & Petersen, D. A. (1997). Sexual attraction toward clients, use of supervision, and prior training: A qualitative study of predoctoral psychology interns. *Journal of Counseling Psychology, 44*(4), 413.

Lamb, D. H., Catanzaro, S. J., & Moorman, A. S. (2003). Psychologists reflect on their sexual relationships with clients, supervisees, and students: Occurrence, impact, rationales and collegial intervention. *Professional Psychology: Research and Practice, 34*(1), 102–107.

LeBlanc, V. R. (2009). The effects of acute stress on performance: Implications for health professions education. *Academic Medicine, 84*(10), S25–S33.

Macapagal, K. R., Janssen, E., Fridberg, D. J., Finn, P. R., & Heiman, J. R. (2011). The effects of impulsivity, sexual arousability, and abstract intellectual ability on men's and women's go/no-go task performance. *Archives of Sexual Behavior, 40*(5), 995–1006.

Malamuth, N. M. (1986). Predictors of naturalistic sexual aggression. *Journal of Personality and Social Psychology, 50*(5), 953.

Mick, T. M., & Hollander, E. (2006). Impulsive-compulsive sexual behavior. *CNS Spectrums, 11*(12), 944–955.

Norris, D. M., Gutheil, T. G., & Strasburger, L. H. (2003). This couldn't happen to me: Boundary problems and sexual misconduct in the psychotherapy relationship. *Psychiatric Services, 54*(4), 517–522.

O'Hara, R. E., Gibbons, F. X., Gerrard, M., Li, Z., & Sargent, J. D. (2012). Greater exposure to sexual content in popular movies predicts earlier sexual debut and increased sexual risk taking. *Psychological Science, 23*(9), 984–993.

Paxton, C., Lovett, J., & Riggs, M. L. (2001). The nature of professional training and perceptions of adequacy in dealing with sexual feelings in psychotherapy: Experiences of clinical faculty. *Ethics & Behavior, 11*(2), 175–189.

Preston, S. D., Buchanan, T. W., Stansfield, R. B., & Bechara, A. (2007). Effects of anticipatory stress on decision making in a gambling task. *Behavioral Neuroscience, 121*(2), 257.

Rodgers, N. M. (2011). Intimate boundaries: Therapists' perception and experience of erotic transference within the therapeutic relationship. *Counselling and Psychotherapy Research, 11*(4), 266–274.

Söchting, I., Fairbrother, N., & Koch, W. J. (2004). Sexual assault of women: Prevention efforts and risk factors. *Violence Against Women, 10*(1), 73–93.

Somer, E., & Saadon, M. (1999). Therapist-client sex: Clients' retrospective reports. *Professional Psychology: Research and Practice, 30*(5), 504–509.

Starcke, K., & Brand, M. (2012). Decision making under stress: A selective review. *Neuroscience & Biobehavioral Reviews, 36*(4), 1228–1248.

Thoreson, R. W., Shaughnessy, P., & Frazier, P. A. (1995). Sexual contact during and after professional relationships: Practices and attitudes of female counselors. *Journal of Counseling & Development, 74*(1), 84–89.

Managing Fantasies   **4**

Sexual fantasies are pleasurable, stimulating, and motivating. They also influence behavior. While the overwhelming majority of sexual fantasies do not lead to problematic sexual behaviors there is no doubt the inverse is true; most sexual activity leading to untoward consequences is preceded by fantasies. Recognizing one's fantasies and knowing how to dissipate their power are necessities in fostering wise sexual decision-making in the clinical realm.

Consider the case of Jessica, a licensed mental health professional working in a small group practice, and her new patient Joseph. Note that some readers may object to the use of an example of a female professional when it is well known that males commit the majority of boundary violations. This is done purposefully so as not to reinforce common stereotypes about the female gender, particularly that they are impervious to sexual temptation and are much more capable of managing arousal. Hamilton and Spruill (1999) remind us that stereotypes about female desire have real-life implications, including failure to address female sexual arousal in education, training, and supervision. The reality is that all genders can be bewildered by sexual arousal, including in the form of fantasy.

A review of Jessica's history presents a number of compounded proximal, distal, and situational risk factors (noted in Chapter 3), particularly life crises and transitions. She separated from her boyfriend of 2 years almost 6 months ago, and her subsequent efforts at online dating have been unsuccessful at best and disasters at worst. She is lonely and still grieving the loss of her former relationship. No less devastating, her mother is being treated for breast cancer, and the early treatment outcomes are not as promising as originally projected. She had little training on sexual attraction during her education and has never considered the possibility that it could occur to her. It is at this period she meets her newest client, Joseph, self-referred for depression and anxiety. He is strikingly handsome, and Jessica finds herself intrigued by her own attraction to him during their work together. During their early sessions,

Jessica discovers he exhibits many of the traits she is desirous of in a romantic partner. As their work together progresses she recognizes she is having fantasies of him, sometimes during sessions with Joseph but more commonly following unsuccessful dating with prospective partners. Sometimes these fantasies are explicitly sexual but more often they are of an idealized romantic nature, including dating Joseph, taking trips together, and raising a family. As she learns more about Joseph's issues, she realizes that in many ways she could be the perfect romantic partner for him; her strengths would balance his limitations and vice versa.

In the case of Jessica, when does fantasy become problematic? Is the mere act of fantasizing about a client a cause for concern? Are sexual fantasies more risky than romantic fantasies? Research is very clear: experiencing sexual or romantic fantasies is not necessarily problematic during mental health treatment; instead they should be expected as part of the process of two people working together in an intimate setting. However they are often the very first indication that a mental health professional has entered the Boundary Violation Cycle and as such must be addressed thoughtfully. The challenge with aforementioned Jessica is not that she is having fantasies of a client (who wouldn't, based on the current dynamics of her life?), the problem is how she is managing them.

The Science of Sexual Fantasies

Sexual fantasy is the most common human sexual experience. Even studies of asexual individuals – commonly defined as individuals not sexually attracted to other people and estimated to comprise 1% of the population – find the majority engage in occasional sexual fantasy (Decker, 2015). The following overview is aggregated by several recurrent themes and questions in research.

What Are Sexual Fantasies?

Research has examined the meaning of fantasies. Are they merely fleeting thoughts that have no particular significance, or do they tell us something meaningful about the person experiencing them? For example, does a married heterosexual male having occasional same-sex fantasies reveal a dormant sexual desire? Many professionals firmly believe fantasies offer more honest insight into a person's sexual desires in comparison to self-reports. Leitenberg and Henning (1995), in their exhaustive review of the research on sexual fantasy stated, "In fantasy one can imagine anything one likes, however unrealistic, without experiencing embarrassment or rejection or societal and legal restrictions. Sexual fantasies, therefore, may provide a unique insight into the different scripts that may underlie sexual behavior" (p. 469).

Other professionals are not so sure and suggest we look at research on dreaming. Studies find that while some dreams are indeed representative of awake-life issues or are a means of expressing unconscious wishes and desires, at other times they are the outcome of the sorting, scanning, and sifting process occurring in the brain while sleeping, in which unnecessary neural connections are eliminated and important ones are strengthened. Sometimes dreams are simply random activity resulting from neurons firing spontaneously in the lower brain that are sent to the cortex, which then tries to make sense of them. In sum, no single theory explains all facets of dreaming. The same holds true for fantasies.

How Are Sexual Fantasies Measured?

Measurement of fantasies remains a problem for the field because people are not forthcoming about personal fantasies they find embarrassing or shameful. Most research on sexual fantasy utilizes self-reporting, typically by asking participants to describe recurring fantasies or by presenting them with a checklist of fantasies on which they indicate those that most occur with them. For example, the "Sexual Fantasy Questionnaire" (Wilson, 1988) asks one to indicate on a scale ranging from 0 (never) to 5 (regularly) how often one fantasizes about activities such as:

- making love out of doors in a romantic setting (e.g., field of flowers, beach at night);
- intercourse with an anonymous stranger;
- watching others have sex; and
- hurting a partner.

Researchers have found alternative methods of measuring sexual fantasy other than self-reporting, including penile plethysmography, which measures changes in blood flow in the penis as males are shown erotic pictures or videos, listen to audio recordings, or read pornographic literature (e.g. Letourneau, 2002). A more recent effort makes use of the Stroop effect, which measures reaction time in naming a color printed in a color not denoted by the name. Spada and Jeglic (2016) used the Stroop task to measure reaction time to neutral words (e.g. "windy"), sexual normative words ("passion") and sexually deviant words ("molest"). Participants were asked to state the word color, while ignoring the meaning of the word. They found that those having deviant sexual interests had slower reaction time to deviant words.

Are There Common Sexual Fantasy Themes?

Generally, fantasies fall into one of two categories. First, memories of past arousing sexual experiences. Second, an imagining of arousing sexual events that haven't happened (and may never happen). Additionally, four themes are prevalent: conventional images of past, present, or imaginary lovers; scenes indicating sexual power and irresistibility; scenes involving varied settings, practices, and positions; and scenes of submission or dominance in which some level of physical force is involved or implied (Leitenberg & Henning, 1995).

Further analysis reveals that males, in comparison to females, engage in fantasies which are sexually graphic (particularly including images of genitals), focus more on a partner's body and on what they want to do to it, involve a variety of partners (including group sex), are impersonal, and demonstrate dominance (Ellis & Symons, 1990). Of course there are women who engage in these very same fantasies just as there are men who engage in the fantasies research ascribes to females (i.e., more passive, more focus on men's interest in their bodies, more romantic, and more emotional).

While existing studies find differences in sexual fantasy based on gender, more cutting edge research examines fantasy at the individual level. Why, for example, does Anthony focus specifically on women's breasts while fantasizing, in contrast to Benjamin, who primarily fantasizes about sexual encounters involving infidelity? Why does Catherine fantasize about a romantic moonlight stroll on the beach with her boyfriend followed by love-making in front of a fireplace, while Dee fantasizes about bondage? There is no doubt that fantasy is hardwired into the human brain. There is also no doubt that the common gender differences in fantasies are based on both socialization and evolution. But why do we have such disparate and idiosyncratic fantasies? The answer to this question it likely multifaceted, but at present one's recurrent sexual fantasy themes seems to be based on exposure to sexual imagery. While some fantasies seem to derive purely from one's imagination, the overwhelming majority arises from what a person has experienced either directly or through what one has heard or read about or seen. The top origins for fantasy appear to be one's own sexual experiences, pornography, modeling by parents and peers, and the general media.

Are There Dangerous Sexual Fantasies?

Studies repeatedly find that our fantasies tend to include a wide gamut of behaviors, many of which, if performed in real life, would have serious complications, including arrest for a sexual offense. Fantasies involving force, coercion, dominance, and power (including rape) are so common that researchers are questioning their longstanding definition of "deviant fantasy." For example, Gee, Devilly, and Ward (2004) found little difference between the fantasy themes of sexual offenders and community samples. Similarly, Bartels and Gannon (2011), in their review of aggression and sexual fantasy, determined that so-called deviant sexual fantasy is so common that we have to question our current conceptualization of the word "deviant." They instead use the descriptor "high-risk sexual fantasy," which they describe as mental imagery whose repeated use can increase the likelihood of engaging in consequential sexual behavior in the presence of certain environmental and/or predisposing factors. In other words, fantasy can be dangerous when it is repetitive and occurring at a time of personal vulnerability *and* with an existing opportunity to act upon it. We will re-visit their definition later in the chapter.

Do Sexual Fantasies Influence Behavior?

Decades of research have led to a comprehensive understanding of the myriad of influences sexual fantasy have on sexual behavior, including sexual offending (e.g., Gee, Ward, Belofastov, & Beech, 2006; Gee, Ward, & Eccleston, 2003; Ward & Beech, 2006).

To start, sexual fantasy is used to purposefully change how one is feeling. This can occur in three ways (see Figure 4.1). First, sexual fantasy is used to alleviate boredom. Second, sexual fantasy is used to alleviate a negative mood (a person experiencing several stressors in their life, such as relationship problems, work problems, and possibly financial concerns may use fantasy to feel better – in effect, fantasizing can temporarily improve mood). Finally, fantasy is used to enhance pre-existing positive feelings. In other words, individuals use sexual fantasy to make a positive event even more exciting. Consider a teenager coming home after a great first date with a new potential romantic partner. The teen in question may masturbate to augment his already existing euphoria. In summary, we purposefully use sexual fantasies to change or elevate our moods.

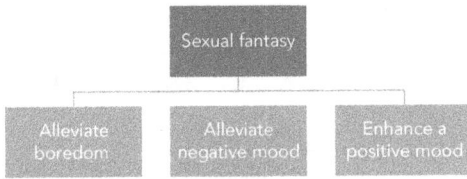

Figure 4.1 Sexual fantasy and emotions
Adapted from Gee, Ward, and Eccleston, 2003

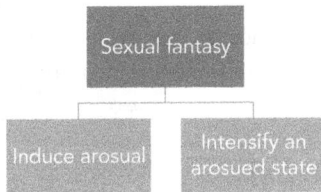

Figure 4.2 Sexual fantasy and sexual arousal
Adapted from Gee, Ward, and Eccleston, 2003

Next, sexual fantasies are also purposefully used to intensify sexual arousal (see Figure 4.2). This occurs in two ways. First, individuals use fantasy to shift from a non-aroused state to one that is prepared for sex; for example, many men with erection problems use fantasy and masturbation to prepare for sexual contact with a partner. Second, fantasy can enhance an existing sexual experience. For example, a woman engaging in sexual activity with her partner may fantasize during the act to make the experience even more exciting. Similarly we can use fantasy to expedite orgasm; a person fantasies during sexual activity to reach a climax quicker. Thus we see that fantasy is voluntarily called upon during sexual activity to prepare for and intensify the experience and to decrease the time it takes to obtain an orgasm.

Finally, sexual fantasy is used to prepare for and rehearse sexual activity (see Figure 4.3). Individuals fantasize about sexual encounters they expect to happen or simply hope will happen. We have all engaged in sexual fantasy in which we mentally rehearse how we will perform and the outcomes we expect. We commonly fantasize about how we can please a sexual partner, often including small details of how we create the "right" environment, our opening sexual moves, how we will respond to a partner's sexual behaviors, etc. Sexual fantasy allows us an opportunity to mentally rehearse sexual activity.

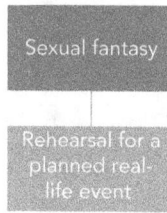

Figure 4.3 Sexual fantasy and goals
Adapted from Gee, Ward, and Eccleston, 2003

In summary, sexual fantasies are not necessarily neutral and involuntary passing thoughts but are instead often purposefully created and called into mind to:

- change how one is feeling;
- initiate and/or intensify sexual experiences; and
- mentally rehearse a desired sexual experience.

Fantasy and Masturbation

Masturbation, an activity that commonly occurs with fantasies, is likewise considered a normative and healthy behavior that occurs throughout the lifespan. An article in the *Journal of Psychology and Human Sexuality* reminds us that throughout history, "[M]asturbation in spite of the ambivalence often expressed about it seems to have been ever present. Pictorial representations of the practice exist from preliterate cultures and references to it can be found in the earliest of writings" (Bullough, 2003, p. 18). A quote in the same journal succinctly summarizes the role of masturbation in human history: "If prostitution is the world's oldest profession, then surely masturbation is the world's oldest avocation" (Pinkerton, Bogart, Cecil, & Abramson, 2003, p. 104). In their exhaustive book *Masturbation: The History of a Great Terror*, Stengers and Van Neck (2001) acquaint modern readers to the prolific eighteenth-century Swiss physician Samuel-Auguste Tissot, whose views on masturbation shaped worldwide cultural perspectives for over 150 years and whose influence is still detected in modern discourse on the topic. Tissot promulgated masturbation as a medical problem leading to:

(1) cloudiness of ideas and sometimes even madness; (2) decay of bodily powers, resulting in coughs, fevers, and consumption; (3) acute pains

in the head, rheumatic pains, and an aching numbness; (4) pimples of the face, suppurating blisters on the nose, breast, and thighs, and painful itchings; (5) eventual weakening of the power of generation as indicated by impotence, premature ejaculation, gonorrhea, priapism, and tumors in the bladder; and (6) disordering of the intestines, resulting in constipation, hemorrhoids, and so forth.

(pp. 65–6)

It wasn't until the 1940s when intrepid sex researcher Alfred Kinsey and his colleagues released their pioneering findings regarding male and female masturbation that the topic began to enter mainstream conversation; they found almost all of the men and more than half of the women interviewed reported having masturbated. It was then that society began to reconsider long-held beliefs regarding masturbation.

Now, more than 75 years later, we have amassed sufficient research on masturbation, including:

- many people learn about their bodies and sexual responsiveness via masturbation;
- it is a safe alternative when there is a risk of a sexually transmitted infection;
- it can help single people who do not have an available partner to maintain sexual functioning and expression; and
- it provides a sexual outlet for individuals when their partners are disinterested in sex or are unavailable.

Masturbation and fantasy are normative behaviors that occur across the lifespan, often occur together, and are an indication of healthy human development.

When Do Fantasies Become High-Risk?

In their interview with predoctoral psychology interns, Ladany et al. (1997) found many reported engaging in sexual fantasies about clients. Do all sexual fantasies of a client indicate problems? Let's be clear at the onset of this section that the goal is not the eradication of fantasy. Sexual fantasizing is part of our human nature and adds immeasurably to the quality of our lives. Additionally, this text will not offer rigid strictures as to what the content of sexual fantasies should or should not be. No fantasy by itself (even when occurring with masturbation) is necessarily "bad," no matter how perverse it might seem to other people. Still, a fantasy can be unhealthy and risky when it moves one closer to committing a sexual act that could have unwanted consequences; or, using the topic of this book, if it leads one to progress along the Boundary Violation Cycle.

Frequency

Several criteria exist to determine whether a fantasy is high-risk or not. First, *high-risk fantasies are frequent and repeated*. A single fantasy – no matter how arousing or disturbing – is not a cause for overreaction. Fantasies occur, and sometimes they contain content that seems contrary to one's beliefs and values. An infrequent or singular sexual fantasy will have marginal impact on sexual decision-making. However, when a fantasy is repeated and frequent, it is time to consider its implications, particularly if it contains material that, if acted upon, could damage one's life (and possibly inflict harm upon another). For example, a woman having a repeated fantasy of making love to her boyfriend on a secluded beach is a very different to a repeated fantasy of making love to a client in the same setting. Repeated fantasies are often signs that specific personal needs are not being met and goals are not being accomplished. The topic of unmet primary goals will be addressed later in Chapter 6.

Current Life Circumstances

The second factor that helps us to determine whether a fantasy is unhealthy or high-risk involves *current life circumstances*. Is one in a setting where a repeated fantasy could actually become reality? A supervisor having repeated fantasies about a famous film celebrity has little chance of living it. In contrast, a repeated sexual fantasy of one of his current graduate students is far more risky. Similarly, the risk level of a male experiencing repeated sexual fantasies of power and domination over others markedly increases when he obtains a promotion to a supervisory position, particularly in a workplace culture supportive of sexist attitudes and the devaluation of females.

Another consideration regarding life circumstances is one's *current emotional state*. Chapter 3 noted that a treatment provider's life crises and life transitions are significant risk factors for a clinical sexual boundary violation. Thus recurrent sexual fantasies of a client occurring during a high-stress period in one's life are particularly risky. Self-control is a finite resource (Sapolsky, 2017), and mental health professionals confronted with sexual attraction to a client might be able to less regulate their behavior based on the amount of stress, problem solving, and need to engage in self-control required for other life predicaments.

Rehearsal and Habituation

Finally, the processes of *rehearsal* and *habituation* evince risk. In criminal justice, an examination of sex offenders shows a consistent finding: many report sexual fantasy preceded their offending, including preparing via fantasy as to how they would both overcome a victim's resistance and minimize detection and consequences. Recall that we all use fantasy, at least on occasion, to mentally prepare for an impending sexual interaction. If a repeated fantasy of a client is evolving into a rehearsal for a desired sexual outcome, there is a reason for concern.

If a person is beginning to include more extreme elements to intensify a fantasy, this too is likely unhealthy and high-risk. As occurs with all activities that lead to a dopamine rush in the brain, repeated engagement necessitates higher amounts of an activity to experience the original amount of pleasure. While one cup of coffee might have kept us going for hours, we now need three for the same burst of energy. A perpetual thrill seeker pursues increasingly dangerous and risky endeavors to obtain the same rush that once came with far less extreme outlets. Fantasy is the same. Repeated use of a particular fantasy lessens its ability to stimulate, and people often begin to include more exotic and/or extreme elements to intensify the experience. If one's fantasies of a client increasingly need to incorporate coercion, force, domination, pain, and/or humiliation in order to achieve satisfaction, this too is propelling one along towards the next step of the Boundary Violation Cycle.

The more of these risk factors a person experiences, the more likely we can label their fantasies as high-risk or, at the least, worrisome (see Figure 4.4). While the majority of sexual fantasies are not going to lead to problematic sexual behaviors, there is no doubt that the reverse is also true; most sexual activity leading to unwanted consequences begins with fantasy reflecting these aforementioned criteria.

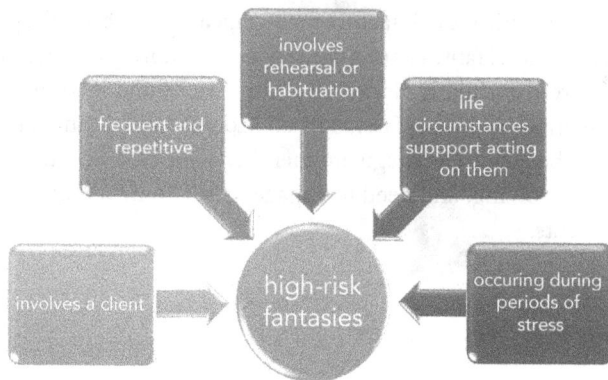

Figure 4.4 The elements of high-risk fantasies

Pornography and Fantasy

Does pornography lead to poor sexual decision-making? Many think it does. In 2016, Utah Governor Gary Herbert called pornography a "public health crisis" and signed two pieces of legislation intended to combat the influence of pornography in his state. In 2018, Florida too followed suit when the state legislature passed a resolution declaring pornography a public health risk.

A 2015 review of studies from seven countries by Wright, Tokunaga, and Kraus determined,

> [T]he accumulated data leave little doubt that, on the average, individuals who consume pornography more frequently are more likely to hold attitudes conducive to sexual aggression and engage in actual acts of sexual aggression than individuals who do not consume pornography or who consume pornography less frequently.
>
> (p. 201)

Pornography also impacts non-aggressive sexual behaviors, including:

- one's romantic partner is often considered less attractive after engaging in porn use;
- erosion of commitment to a current relationship;
- development of positive attitudes towards infidelity; and
- unrealistic beliefs about sexual activity – sexual activity in pornography is typically depicted as spontaneous, complication and responsibility free, and always leading to orgasm. Individuals are sorely disappointed when this does not consistently occur in real life.

Finally, as to the longstanding argument that pornography might have a cathartic effect in which one's mounting libido can be relieved by use of pornography, the verdict is in: there is no evidence that pornography is cathartic and reduces risk; instead, it is associated with an increased risk of acting on one's fantasies.

In sum, watching pornography depicting one's high-risk fantasy is likely to promote progression to the next stage of the Boundary Violation Cycle.

Managing Fantasies

Fantasy is the gateway to behavior. Rarely does it directly lead to overt sexual behavior, but it instead facilitates the process of moving to the next step along the Boundary Violation Cycle. Each step forward on this cycle increase the risk of a bad sexual decision. What then should we do when we recognize that we are experiencing a repeated sexual fantasy that, if engaged in real life, would have disastrous consequences?

- Acknowledge that a strong and/or repeated sexual fantasy is likely an indicator that a person is unfulfilled in certain domains in one's life. Chapter 6 will guide readers through the process of identifying their idiosyncratic primary motivating factors/life drives, which, when blocked or stymied, lead to an increase in fantasies in which they are acted out. For example, a person who prizes autonomy may begin to fantasize about behaviors involving power over other people when in real life he or she is constricted in a micromanaging workplace or involved with a jealous and over-controlling romantic partner. Once these blocked needs have been identified, a person can than begin to formulate a plan to satisfy them.
- Be purposeful in fantasy, porn use, and masturbation imagery. Sexual fantasies, particularly combined with masturbation and/or pornography, are reinforcing. We obtain pleasure from them, or we obtain relief from a negative emotion. Still, we have the option to forgo particular fantasies that increase the likelihood of moving us along the Boundary Violation Cycle. In short, refrain from fantasizing about sexual scenarios and watching pornography that meet the criteria discussed throughout this chapter. We have a choice as to what we fantasize about. We could have a different sexual fantasy (or several fantasies) every day of our lives and come nowhere close to exhausting the diversity of fantasy possibilities.
- Seek Supervision/Consultation. Recall that most mental health professionals do not reveal their sexual attraction or fantasies regarding a client

to a supervisor due to embarrassment or fear of repercussion. Yet it is essential. Disclosure is even more onerous for those professionals lacking or having no access to a supervisor, such as individuals engaged in private practice, one of the noted risk factors associated with poor clinical decision-making regarding sexual matters. For these individuals it is necessary to seek out the support of a colleague. What matters is that a professional has a trusted support person who recognizes a particular fantasy of a client is troubling, problematic, or unwanted; knows the legal, ethical, personal, and therapeutic repercussions of acting on a fantasy of a client; and can offer sound non-judgmental guidance.

Conclusions

The first-step towards a perilous sexual outcome is fantasy. Sexual fantasizing is a commonplace activity and, in spite of our morals and values about the act, is not necessarily a cause for alarm, even when it depicts images that are contrary to the type of person we want to be and the lives we want to live. Fantasies become high-risk when they meet specific criteria, which include:

- frequent and repeated portrayal of illegal, unethical, or personally reprehensible behaviour, which could lead to destructive consequences for oneself or others;
- occurences during times of high stress in one's life;
- the possibility exists that, with planning, the fantasy could become reality;
- imagined rehearsals for risky sexual acts or incorporating increasingly extreme elements to intensify the pleasure and satisfaction they offer.

Fantasies rarely lead to direct engagement in behavior in the real world. Instead, they propel a person to the next step of the Boundary Violation Cycle. Unfortunately, the more one advances along the cycle the more challenging it is to exit it and the more likely one is to engage in a consequential sexual act. The best approach to high-risk fantasies is to stop engaging in them; the number of fantasy scenario substitutes is unlimited. Concurrently, identify why these high fantasies are occurring at this point in one's life. What are the underlying unresolved issues driving them? Finally, seek professional guidance, support, and supervision.

Summary

- Fantasy is the gateway to behavior. Most sexual activity leading to untoward consequences is preceded by fantasy.
- Research on fantasy has come to several conclusions:
  - sexual fantasy is the most common human sexual experience;
  - no single theory explains all facets of fantasizing;
  - fantasies typically fall into one of two categories. First, memories of past arousing sexual experiences. Second, an imagining of arousing sexual events that haven't happened or may never happen; and
  - fantasies involving force, coercion, dominance, and power are so common that researchers are questioning their longstanding definition of "deviant fantasy."
- Fantasies can be purposefully created and called into mind to:
  - change how one is feeling;
  - initiate and/or intensify sexual experiences; and
  - mentally rehearse a desired sexual experience.
- No fantasy by itself is necessarily high-risk. A fantasy is unhealthy and risky when it leads one to progress along the Boundary Violation Cycle.
- Several criteria exist to determine whether a fantasy is high-risk for mental health professionals:
  - fantasies involving a client;
  - fantasies that occur frequently and are repeated;
  - fantasies involving content that could become reality based on current life circumstances;
  - fantasies that occur during a period of stress, likely life crises or transitions; and
  - the fantasy process involves rehearsal and/or habituation.
- Watching pornography depicting one's high-risk fantasy is likely to promote progression to the next stage of the Boundary Violation Cycle.

- There are three recommendations for dealing with a professionals fantasies in clinical settings:
  - acknowledge that a strong and/or repeated sexual fantasy is likely an indicator that a person is unfulfilled in certain prime areas in one's life;
  - be purposeful in fantasy, porn use, and masturbation imagery; and
  - discuss with a colleague or supervisor.

References

Bartels, R. M., & Gannon, T. A. (2011). Understanding the sexual fantasies of sex offenders and their correlates. *Aggression and Violent Behavior, 16*(6), 551–561.

Bullough, V. L. (2003). Masturbation: A historical overview. *Journal of Psychology & Human Sexuality, 14*(2–3), 17–33.

Decker, J.S. (2015). *The invisible orientation: An introduction to asexuality.* New York: Skyhorse Publishing.

Ellis, B. J., & Symons, D. (1990). Sex differences in sexual fantasy: An evolutionary psychological approach. *Journal of Sex Research, 27*(4), 527–555.

Gee, D., Ward, T., Belofastov, A., & Beech, A. (2006). The structural properties of sexual fantasies for sexual offenders: A preliminary model. *Journal of Sexual Aggression, 12*(3), 213–226.

Gee, D., Ward, T., & Eccleston, L. (2003). The function of sexual fantasies for sexual offenders: A preliminary model. *Behaviour Change, 20*(1), 44–60.

Gee, D. G., Devilly, G. J., & Ward, T. (2004). The content of sexual fantasies for sexual offenders. *Sexual Abuse: A Journal of Research and Treatment, 16*(4), 315–331.

Hamilton, J. C., & Spruill, J. (1999). Identifying and reducing risk factors related to trainee–Client sexual misconduct. *Professional Psychology: Research and Practice, 30*(3), 318–327.

Ladany, N., O'brien, K. M., Hill, C. E., Melincoff, D. S., Knox, S., & Petersen, D. A. (1997). Sexual attraction toward clients, use of supervision, and prior training: A qualitative study of predoctoral psychology interns. *Journal of Counseling Psychology, 44*(4), 413–424.

Leitenberg, H., & Henning, K. (1995). Sexual fantasy. *Psychological Bulletin, 117*(3), 469.

Letourneau, E. J. (2002). A comparison of objective measures of sexual arousal and interest: Visual reaction time and penile plethysmography. *Sexual Abuse: A Journal of Research and Treatment, 14*(3), 203–219.

Pinkerton, S. D., Bogart, L. M., Cecil, H., & Abramson, P. R. (2003). Factors associated with masturbation in a collegiate sample. *Journal of Psychology & Human Sexuality, 14*(2–3), 103–121.

Sapolsky, R. M. (2017). *Behave: The biology of humans at our best and worst.* New York: Penguin.

Spada, A. H., & Jeglic, E. L. (2016). A cognitive-based indicator of deviant sexual interest: Concurrent validation of the stroop task. *Journal of Sexual Aggression, 22*(2), 246–262.

Stengers, J., & Van Neck, A. (2001). *Masturbation: The history of a great terror* (pp. 65–66). New York: Palgrave.

Ward, T., & Beech, A. (2006). An integrated theory of sexual offending. *Aggression and Violent Behavior, 11*(1), 44–63.

Wilson, G. D. (1988). Measurement of sex fantasy. *Sexual and Marital Therapy, 3*(1), 45–55.

Wright, P. J., Tokunaga, R. S., & Kraus, A. (2015). A meta-analysis of pornography consumption and actual acts of sexual aggression in general population studies. *Journal of Communication, 66*(1), 183–205.

Choosing

5

Talking Ourselves into (and out of) Sexual Predicaments

Sexual fantasies and romantic attraction to clients are common occurrences, and mental health professionals have a choice as to how they deal with these experiences. They can be proactively addressed, ignored with hope and belief that they are inconsequential and will soon dissipate, or, in the worst-case scenario, their influence can be purposefully amplified moving one even closer to a sexual boundary violation.

Let's return to Jessica, who was introduced in Chapter 4. At this point in her work with Joseph she recognizes that her sexual attraction to him is influencing treatment. Not only does she continue to have sexual and romantic fantasies, but also she has been more self-disclosing than she is with any other client. These disclosures have been of marginal importance, such as sharing a film she saw during the past week or letting Joseph know to her surprise that they are both fond of the same band that will be touring soon in their city. She also purposefully tidies herself up before her session with Joseph, including applying make-up and brushing her hair. Jessica has considered discussing her attraction with a colleague, but is embarrassed and fearful; they would likely want her to modify her approach, and, quite frankly, this would necessitate a change in how she works with Joseph, who seems to be responding to treatment so very well. An even worse scenario is that a colleague or supervisor might suggest transferring Joseph to another clinician. Yet they both really enjoy their work together.

We see that Jessica made and continues to make choices. She chooses to continue engaging in fantasies of her client. She chooses to engage in self-disclosure of a non-therapeutic nature. She chooses to avoid supervision or consultation about her attraction. During the *choosing* phase of the Boundary Violation Cycle a clinician makes decisions as to whether he will continue along the path approaching a violation or make efforts to avoid this progression.

Avoidance and Approach Goals

One of the most influential theories in sex offender research is Ward and Hudson's (1998) self-regulation model, which argues that once an individual recognizes the presence of inappropriate or high-risk arousal they make a choice as to what can and should be done about it. In general, there are two options: approach or avoidance. Clinicians, upon recognizing that arousal, attraction, and fantasy are becoming increasingly powerful and/or distracting, must make a choice as to how to manage it, either deciding to move towards a goal of acting on sexual desire, typically by initiating non-sexual boundary crossings, or making efforts to forestall it and, in the best-case scenario, learning about themselves and increasing clinical competence through the experience.

Avoidance Goals

Clinicians, recognizing the consequences of acting on sexual desire occurring within the clinical realm, can and do successfully manage attraction to a client as well as develop improved professional competence through the experience. Martin, Godfrey, Meekums, and Madill (2011) interviewed practicing mental health professionals about their experiences of sexual attraction in therapy. The authors then formulated a model describing the process by which they managed this arousal. Clinicians start by *noting* their attraction to a client, including unease, anxiety, feeling "warmer" towards the person, or even an inchoate recognition that something is different in interactions with this client. During the second stage – *facing up to it personally* – clinicians acknowledge to themselves that they are attracted to a client, which is often accompanied by embarrassment and shame. Clinicians acknowledge fantasizing about a client or making efforts to avoid thinking about the person. *Reflecting, processing, and managing* – the third stage – finds clinicians contemplating on the attraction, considering the implications of the situation, and examining its possible meaning, including their vulnerabilities and current life dissatisfactions. It is at this stage a clinician accepts the impossibility of a romantic or sexual relationship and processes the feelings of loss this entails. During the final stage – *formulating and working for the client's benefit* – the clinician also considers whether their attraction is representative of similar interactions in a client's life and how to incorporate this into the therapy process.

Luca and Boyden (2014) also interviewed mental health professionals and found attraction to a client could lead to improved therapeutic outcomes. Some reported attraction led them to seek information on attraction, engage in personal insight work, talk to supervisors about the experience, and learn how to better self-regulate the tension, discomfort, and excitement that sexual attraction entails. It also led them to formulate methods of using the attraction to facilitate the therapy experience, particularly the use of normalizing attraction and being able to breach the topic with a client with "non-shaming delicacy" (p. 203) when the latter presented with attraction to the professional.

The two aforementioned studies demonstrate that arousal and attraction can be used to therapeutic advantage; clinicians actively use reflection, processing, and consultation to avoid acting on sexual attraction. A second but less salubrious avoidance method is also found in the Luca and Boyden (2014) study. One subset of clinicians reported feeling uncomfortable, unsure, and even frightened about their attraction to a client. These individuals responded by becoming more authoritative, firm, intellectualizing, and disengaging in sessions. Their efforts at over-controlling sessions enable them to avoid acting on attraction but also damage a relationship with a likely confused client; it also stymied opportunity for growth in self-regulation and learning skills for managing arousal in the future. Some professionals use other ineffective coping strategies, such as speaking to friends about attraction but who are unable to offer sound clinical guidance instead of broaching the topic with colleagues or a supervisor; such solutions are often inadequate for coping with clinical attraction. Others use maladaptive coping mechanisms that inadvertently increase the likelihood of acting on arousal. For example, a clinician may engage in masturbation involving a fantasy of a client, which may temporarily lessen libido but actually reinforces an association between the client and sexual arousal. Alcohol and use of other intoxicants, a common self-management strategy, may lead to disinhibition.

Finally, and an unfortunately common response to clinical arousal, is an avoidant-passive approach (Ward & Hudson, 1998), in which professionals ignore the problem and wait for it to go away, either by waiting for attraction to decrease on its own or for a client to leave treatment. According to Bickley and Beech (2002) individuals following this route do not know how to proactively manage their arousal, are unassertive, and have an external locus of control.

The work summarized above demonstrates that sexual attraction can facilitate the treatment process as well as a professional's development when approached correctly, which typically encompasses use of supervision or therapy for oneself. However, this approach is often elided in favor of the over-controlling or avoidant-passive methods, which may be less embarrassing and clinically taxing but also negate therapist development and can harm a clinical relationship.

Approach Goals: Predatory Clinicians

The Ward and Hudson self-regulation model (1998) acknowledges that some individuals purposefully and even relentlessly seek out sexual activity that victimizes others. All existing typologies of clinicians engaging in sexual boundary violations acknowledge their presence, typically referring to them as predatory. While the majority of clinicians who engage in a boundary violation do so only once, predatory clinicians amass multiple victims throughout their professional careers.

Predatory clinicians utilize grooming and seduction to obtain their goals of sexual contact with a client without detection. The concept of grooming was developed through research and clinical work with those offending against children and their victims, and Craven, Brown, and Gilchrist (2006) formulated a definition encompassing a myriad of research findings occurring since the topic was originally introduced into the literature decades earlier. According to the authors, grooming is "a process by which a person prepares a child, significant adults and the environment for the abuse of this child. Specific goals include gaining access to the child, gaining the child's compliance and maintaining the child's secrecy to avoid disclosure" (p. 297). Grooming is not a singular event and can extend for an indefinite period of time. Williams, Elliott, and Beech (2013) state the process "can develop over the duration of hours, days, months, or even years, depending on the needs (and the patience) of the offender" (p. 137).

Grooming typically has three goals. First, it is a planned and purposeful effort to overcome the resistance of a possible victim, typically by establishing an ostensibly trustworthy, safe, and intimate relationship. Second, there is a gradual sexualization of the relationship. For example, many offenders desensitize a child by initiating physical contact through stroking a child's head or patting their back and then gradually progressing to more intimate forms of contact. The offending adult may also introduce seemingly innocuous conversations about dating or boyfriends/girlfriends, which then, over time, becomes more explicitly sexual. Third, there is a goal of proactively minimizing disclosure of the offense afterwards. Offenders against children often make the latter reliant on them for praise, financial support, and attention. They can psychologically manipulate a child to believe he or she is responsible for the sexual act. If an offender recognizes discomfort or distress in an intended victim during the grooming process, they can stop the process or, more likely, devise a more strategic method of continuing the grooming.

A similar process occurs with adult victims and is frequently titled "seduction." Tanner and Brake (2013) found that offenders against adults engage in a three-step process prior to offending. First, the offender bonds by formation of a supportive relationship with a vulnerable adult, often one who is lonely and isolated, has low self-esteem or self-valuation, or is attempting to escape intolerable living conditions, such as abuse, oppression, and/or poverty. The second step of the process is fostering increasing reliance on the offender while simultaneously promoting isolation and estrangement from other possible supports. Finally, the offender gradually sexualizes their relationship or coerces them into sexual activity.

Grooming and seduction occur on multiple levels. While research highlights the process of directly grooming victims, others have noted offenders groom others in victims' lives. Grooming of parents, siblings, and other responsible adults is necessary for offenders' ultimate goal of sexual contact with a child. They often present themselves as caring and trustworthy adults who can be left alone in the company of children; this valued reputation also makes it less likely that an accusation against them will be believed. van Dam (2001) reports that offenders are frequently charming, very helpful, and have insider status. Offenders against adults often engage in a similar process of establishing positions held in high regard and in which they are sought for advice due to their social position, such as clergy, social worker, or therapist. They also often present as deeply concerned about the welfare of others and as low risk for engaging in sexual coercion and manipulation.

The planning of predatory mental health workers very much follows the patterns noted above. They enter workplaces with the intent of gaining access to new victims – whether adults, adolescents, or children – target one (or several), and strategize a grooming/seduction process to accomplish this outcome and that minimizes the chance of victim disclosure or believability.

Other Approach Strategies

Most professionals engaging romantically or sexually with a client are not predatory. Many sexual boundary crossings, for example, occur after a professional has fallen in love with a client. These individuals typically present with a series of earlier noted proximal and distal risk factors, are triggered by a particular client, and are experiencing a life crisis or transition. They feel guilty about their attraction, recognize its consequences, but are nonetheless compelled to act on it, often through seductive means and escalating boundary crossings. In no way are they predatory as the word is commonly understood since there will likely be no additional victims.

Ward and Hudson's (1998) self-regulation model identified one final pathway by which a person moves closer to acting on deviant sexual desire, the approach-automatic pathway. Similar to predatory clinicians, these individuals have a desire to act on their arousal, but, in contrast, do not make active plans to offend. There is no grooming or seduction. They instead respond to situational cues and passively allow circumstances to lead to a boundary violation. This often occurs in a scenario in which a client makes their attraction to their treatment professional known. The clinician, also attracted, passively allows the situation to advance, making no efforts to stop or promote a boundary crossing. Individuals using this approach later claim a boundary violation "just happened."

Summary of the Avoidance and Approach Goals

Upon recognizing sexual attraction to a client, clinicians have two overall approaches as to how to proceed. In general, they can make efforts to avoid further inflaming their attraction or they can choose to promote further sexual and romantic involvement. For those who choose to avoid exacerbation, one option is reflection, processing of attraction, and clinical consultation. However more common is the use of over-controlling and overcompensation in treatment or passively avoiding the topic and waiting for it to ameliorate on its own. For those who decide to advance towards a boundary violation, we find three general patterns. First, we have predatory clinicians. Second, we have clinicians, most often those who have fallen in love with a client, who want to build a relationship. And, finally, there is a group that passively allows circumstances to dictate how their attraction will play out.

The predatory, lovesick, and approach-automatic pathways inevitably lead to the next phase of the Boundary Violation Cycle, but even those using an avoidance approach will often use maladaptive or ineffective strategies to stop their progression. They truly don't want to engage in a boundary violation but do not have the resources, knowledge, or skills to halt their progress, or use counterproductive interventions that unintentionally move them further along the cycle. Sexual arousal and attraction to a client is best managed in a supervisor relationship or consultation, but this option is unlikely to occur.

Influences on Choosing

There is no monolithic or quintessential depiction of a boundary-violating clinician. Some may be psychopathic predators. Others may be new to the field, have little formal training on sexual self-management, and are supervised by individuals who steadfastly avoid the topic due to their own discomfort. Some clinicians may be undergoing tumultuous life transitions or crises and are fairly isolated in their work. Regardless of their specific circumstances, all engage in sexual decision-making, with an outcome of either moving closer to or further away from a sexual boundary violation.

Decision-making regarding arousal and attraction in clinical practice *seems* easy; after all, a logical cost-analysis weighing the advantages and repercussions of sexual involvement with a client leads to a conclusion that it is too damaging for all involved, including collateral victims such as family members, colleagues, an organization's reputation, and even the field in general. Still it occurs, and this section will describe a myriad of often-unacknowledged obstacles that hinder optimal decision-making.

The Limits to Logic

Unfortunately, humans are not quite as good at logical problem solving as we like to believe, and the ability of situational factors to override common sense is increasingly acknowledged. Nobel laureate in economics Herbert Simon (1979) determined that instead of making optimal choices, humans tend to engage in *satisficing*, which is seeking solutions that satisfy and suffice. He proposed we are not completely rational in our decision-making but are instead impacted by information processing capacity, subconscious cues, and situational factors. In Simon's terms, humans have limitations in rational problem solving, which he termed *bounded rationality*.

The brain uses many short cuts when engaging in problem solving that do not necessarily lead to optimal decisions. For example, the availability heuristic predicts that we make decisions based on how easy it is to recall relevant examples. We may determine that air travel is more risky if we can easily recall a number of recent airline disasters. Another cognitive bias is the sunk-cost fallacy, which predicts that we will continue along a particular path of action no matter how costly simply because we have already invested in it. The confirmation bias too is well founded in research and finds we interpret evidence that support existing beliefs. Even physical states influence decision-making; bad tastes and smells lead people to be more judgmental (Haidt, 2012).

These examples indicate that we do not necessarily make important decisions based on logic but rather unconsciously utilize cognitive short cuts, biases, and even bodily states to determine a course or outcome. Also, these limitations cannot easily be overcome. Haidt (2012) for example determined that the confirmation bias is "ineradicable." He asks,

> How hard could it be to teach students to look at the other side, to look for evidence against their favored view? Yet, in fact, it's very hard and nobody has yet found a way to do it. It's hard because the confirmation bias is built-in feature [of the brain]....
>
> (p. 105)

The Limits to Self-Control

Self-control and will power can change through a week, a day, or even an hour. While some individuals habitually demonstrate self-control deficits, we all experience lapses in will power based on circumstances in our lives. Self-control is a finite resource (Sapolsky, 2017). Ingenious experimental studies (e.g., Muraven, Tice, & Baumeister, 1998; Vohs et al., 2008) find engaging in self-regulation leads to depleted ability to engage in optimal subsequent efforts. Like other bodily capacities such as strength and energy, self-regulation ability can become temporarily exhausted.

Building upon existing literature on self-regulation, the impact of tiredness on sexual-decision making has recently been explored. It is already known that tired individuals are less likely to self-regulate in general, to engage in more risk-taking, and to be more emotionally reactive (Palmer & Alfano, 2017). Few studies though have directly examined the impact of tiredness on sexual behavior, but Millar, Starks, Rendina, and Parsons (2018) determined tiredness increases sexual desire in males and engagement in risky behaviors. This impact of tiredness on sexual decision-making remains a pertinent area for future research.

Arousal and Sexual Decision-Making

Sexual arousal too impacts decision-making. Consider the oversexualization effect, which could partially explain why males engage in far more sexual boundary violations than females. Abbey's (1982) groundbreaking work on this topic determined males tend to judge women as being seductive and promiscuous in even neutral interactions. In general, men see the world in far more sexual terms than women. Decades of research, including naturalistic studies, interactions between the sexes in laboratory settings, and responses to vignettes, photographs, and filmed depictions find the same result (Jacques-Tiura, Abbey, & Parkhill 2007). In essence, men, far more than women, are prone to perceive sexual intent when it does not actually exist, and some posit this is a factor in sexual aggression and coercion (e.g., Farris, Treat, Viken, & McFall, 2008). While the oversexualization effect is unlikely to lead to a sexual boundary violation on its own, in combination with other risk factors noted throughout this text (e.g., self-regulation difficulties; sexual compulsion) the risk in increased.

Ariely and Loewenstein (2006) asked males to masturbate to an aroused state and then to answer questions about how appealing they find a wide range of sexual stimuli and activities, their willingness to engage in morally questionable behavior in order to obtain sexual gratification, and, finally, their willingness to engage in unsafe sex. The researchers found arousal acts an "amplifier" in that it leads males to find a much wider range of activities as sexually appealing in comparison to when they are not aroused. Also, males reported more willingness to engage in risky sexual behaviors and use questionable and even illegal behaviors to increase the likelihood of obtaining sex (e.g., falsely tell a woman he loved her; encourage a woman to drink alcohol, or furtively give a woman a drug). Even more concerning, the authors determined we are often unaware of the insidious impact of arousal on decision-making and they enjoin us to remember that it is difficult while in an unaroused state to appreciate and recall just how powerful arousal can be. Thus we castigate professionals who engage in poor sexual decision-making while discounting that we too could act the same way in an arousing and possibly compromising situation.

Skakoon-Sparling, Cramer, and Shuper (2016) expanded studies of arousal and decision-making to include females. Using sexually explicit and neutral video clips, they found men and women reporting more arousal described more intent to engage in risky sexual behavior as well as presenting with lowered inhibitions and impaired decision-making. Both genders were vulnerable to the impact of sexual arousal on decisions about sexual behaviors.

In sum, studies clearly point out that arousal impacts decision-making. It is yet unclear though exactly how this occurs. Does arousal deplete available self-control resources or make executive functioning abilities less accessible? One hypothesis is borrowed from the substance-use research: alcohol myopia. Myopia – a descriptor for nearsightedness – aptly describes the experiences individuals have while intoxicated. Introduced into the literature by Steele and Josephs (1990), it postulates that substance use: (1) restricts the range of cues one can perceive in a situation (when a person is intoxicated he cannot attend to and encode available cues, both internal and external); and (2) reduces the ability to process and extract meaning from the cues and information that can be perceived. Alcohol myopia is characterized by an attention bias towards salient situational cues that "strongly motivate a response that, if one were sober, would be inhibited by further access to other cues and meanings" (p. 931). Sexual arousal seems to act in the same way; it creates a form of tunnel vision in which the proximal goals of sexual gratification and pleasure temporarily override consideration about likely consequences.

Internal Dialogue and Self-Talk

In the 1960s Aaron Beck, a pioneer in the cognitive behavioral approach, originally set about evaluating the psychoanalytic approaches to treatment of depression fully expecting them to be successful. He experienced confusion in finding the opposite; many clients experienced frequent and automatic patterns of negative thinking, often about themselves, their futures, and the world in general that were not amenable to psychoanalysis. Decades of research have built upon and elaborated on these findings, particularly the role of irrational thoughts and interpretations. Burns (1989) delineated several prevalent cognitive distortions that are targeted in treatment. The following examples represent only a partial list of recognized cognitive distortions.

- **All-or-nothing thinking/black-and-white thinking** – Using this distortion people interpret events in terms of extremes – something is either fantastic or awful.
- **Overgeneralization** – One instance or example is generalized to an overall pattern.
- **Mind reading** – The inaccurate belief that we know what another person is thinking.
- **Catastrophizing or minimization** – This distortion involves exaggerating the importance or meaning of things or minimizing the importance or meaning of things.
- **Personalization** – This distortion involves assigning blame to oneself when no such responsibility exists.

The power of self-talk is a cornerstone in all cognitive therapy models, and many common mental health problems such as anxiety, depression, and substance use are treated with cognitive approaches with great success. These models conclude that we interact with and respond to the world based on mental representations of it. If these representations are inaccurate or distorted our resulting emotions and behavior are likely faulty and even counterproductive. Cognitive models of therapy assist individuals to recognize their idiosyncratic maladaptive self-talk and learn to think more realistically and productively.

Over time the field of sexual offending treatment began to incorporate cognitive distortions into their protocols. Finkelhor's (1984) early model of sexual abuse proposed that overcoming "internal barriers" (i.e., knowing that what one is doing is wrong) is a precondition for offending. A person progresses towards an offense by using cognitive distortions and faulty self-talk that enables them to: (1) get past the fear of getting caught; (2) decide that a victim's feelings don't matter; and (3) ignore the recognition that what one is doing is wrong. Decades later, the role of self-talk and cognitive distortions is now a foundation in conceptualizing offending and used prolifically throughout treatment. In their comprehensive assessment protocol for adult sexual offenders, for example, Carich and Adkerson (1995) measure thinking errors typically used by an offender, including:

- Predicting the future – "I know this is wrong, but I can get away with it."
- Justification – "I deserve this" or "If she would had just said 'no' more forcibly I would have stopped."
- Jumping to conclusions – "She smiled at me. I know she is attracted to me."

Lamb, Catanzaro, and Moorman (2003) surveyed practicing psychologists who had engaged in prohibited sexual relationships with clients, supervisees, and students. When asked to describe their decision-making process, three general patterns were noted. First, 40% reported a *no harm, thus I proceed* distortion as depicted in rationalizations such as: "no harm to the other person;" "the therapy relationship was over, no dual role;" or "time since termination was sufficient." The second error, *consulted and negotiated*, was described in 32% of responses and illustrated by statements such as: "clarified through peer consultation and then proceeded;" "we agreed that the formal relationship would not occur again;" or "I discussed relationship characteristics with the other person and kept clear roles related to the new relationship." The third category of explanation, *continued although I knew the behavior was problematic and/or unethical*, was evident in 28% of responses and depicted in the following statements: "I saw the relationship as personally problematic but I continued;" or "I saw my behavior as violating ethical standards, but I continued." In addition, approximately one half of the individuals indicated that they stopped the professional relationship in order to proceed with the sexual relationship, a common behavior in professional sexual boundary violations used to give a misleading patina of credibility to the behavior.

Cognitive Schemas

Offender treatment also attempts to correct problematic cognitive schemas and underlying – and often implicit – beliefs that facilitate offending. Child abusers often believe that children are sexual beings and that sex does not cause harm to them (Ward & Keenan, 1999). Rapists often believe that heterosexual encounters are inherently adversarial and that women should be sexually receptive to men's needs (Polaschek & Ward, 2002). In an early article on boundary violating physicians, Abel, Osborn, and Warberg (1995) wrote that professionals interpret sexual contact with a client as a voluntary activity between two consenting adults and having nothing to do with a patient–physician relationship. The role of cognitive schemas has belatedly become a topic of investigation regarding boundary-violating clinicians. McNulty, Ogden, and Warren (2013) began their article by stating their belief that the majority of sexual boundary violations are not the work of predatory clinicians but rather, "given the right circumstances, most mental health practitioners could be vulnerable to breaching ethical rules" (p. 191). They interviewed mental health professionals who had been professionally censured for sexual boundary violations and found a theme of *neutralization of a client's "patientness."* Clinicians did not begin a relationship until they believed a patient's psychological issues had been resolved. At this point power balances were ostensibly dissolved, professional boundaries could be more lax, and a conventional relationship was seen as possible. In short, a reduction in mental health symptoms was a pre-condition for boundary crossings.

Summary of Influences on Choosing

This section elucidated the obstacles to optimal sexual decision-making, in which the best outcomes for a client and the professional are carefully scrutinized and considered. Instead, due to the influences described in this chapter, professionals make poor sexual decisions that could have ramifications for their entire lives. These influences include limitations to logical thinking and self-control; the impact of arousal on decision-making; faulty self-talk, cognitive distortions, and problematic implicit schemas. One of these is sufficient to complicate logical problem solving, but in situations involving arousal to a client, we experience an often-overpowering conflux of multiple factors.

Enhancing Sexual Decision-Making

At some point a mental health professional recognizes that once-ephemeral fantasies of a client have become more intrusive. Maybe they are more frequent or combined with masturbation. Maybe the professional is beginning to compare an idealized patient to a current and dissatisfying romantic relationship partner. They may even treat the client with more friendliness, concern, and openness but have not yet transgressed any specific boundaries. This recognition – which might develop gradually or suddenly appear in a moment of insight – necessitates a choice as to how to proceed. A clinician can move towards or away from a foreseeable sexual boundary violation, or they may stolidly allow circumstances to determine an outcome.

Moving away from a boundary violation is the best course of action, but the obstacles to optimal decision-making noted in this chapter – self-deception, arousal, permissive self-talk, cognitive distortions, faulty schemas, and depleted self-regulatory ability – lead many clinicians to rationalize and justify moving instead onto the next phase of the Boundary Violation Cycle, and thus become one step closer to an actual violating behavior.

For clinicians who are finding it increasingly difficult to refute the rationalizations and justifications urging a boundary violation as well as bolster realistic concerns about its impact on a client and themselves, three interventions are supported:

- First, engage in supervision or honest consultation with a colleague. As this chapter has explained, we are able to deceive ourselves, which is then compounded by our poor competence with logic and problem solving. Sexual arousal too impacts how we weigh costs and benefits. A trusted third party is often the only way to circumnavigate the cognitive traps that can otherwise ensnare us.
- The second approach is to picture the true narrative arc of a desired boundary violation. Professionals tend to focus their attention on the beginning short-term rapturous moments of a boundary violation, such as satisfying

sexual activity, a meaningful relationship, and the joys and infatuation of a new romance. They rarely consider the long-term impact such as the need to maintain secrecy, the self-recrimination that arises, and the harm that could befall all touched by the event, including collateral victims. Focus then on the long-term meaning of a boundary violation rather than the temporary pleasure it will bring at its beginning.

- Finally, for those professionals whose struggle to avoid progressing along the Boundary Violation Cycle is too overwhelming or who have convinced themselves that this egregious behavior is acceptable, the only intervention is to escape. Stop seeing the client, even if only temporarily and until one can discuss this with a supervisor or colleague. Rarely would lying to a client be justified, but in a critical moment such as this, informing them that a family member is ill or has died or whatever excuse comes to mind and will allow several weeks distance from the patient is the only viable course of action. Explanations can come later, and the therapeutic relationship can be salvaged, but a sexual boundary violation, in contrast, is irrevocable.

Conclusions

Clinicians can move towards or away from a professional sexual boundary violation; they make choices leading them in one direction or the other. Even refusing to make a decision and allowing fate to determine the outcome is still a decision. In choosing to move away from an actual violation, professionals can use their arousal for therapeutic growth. Through processing their arousal and attractions, clinicians can recognize unmet needs (to be addressed in the next chapter) and current life dissatisfactions that lead them to be vulnerable to future incidents of sexual attraction in clinical settings. It can also assist clinicians to improve self-regulatory abilities. Finally, it can be used diagnostically to expand and elaborate upon problematic sexual issues and themes that may recurrently play out in clients' lives. However, many will make counterproductive choices due to shame, confusion, self-confidence, and/or the unwillingness to forego the compelling lure of eroticized clinical interactions. The challenges to rational decision-making noted in this chapter no doubt impact this decision, including self-deception, arousal, permissive self-talk, cognitive distortions, and depleted self-regulatory ability. In the end, most professionals choose to wait attraction out while telling themselves, "I can stop this at any time I want." However, the longer one remains in the cycle, the more difficult it is to extricate oneself.

Summary

- Mental health professionals have a choice as to how they deal with attraction, arousal, and fantasy concerning a client.
- Professionals typically use either an avoidance or approach style when dealing with attraction to a client.
- Avoidance methods:
  - Those utilizing the recommended avoidance style talk to supervisors about the experience, learn how to better self-regulate the tension, discomfort, and excitement sexual attraction entails, and to formulate methods of using the attraction to facilitate the therapy experience.
  - A less successful avoidance style is becoming over-controlling in sessions.
  - A similarly less successful avoidant style is the avoidant-passive approach in which one waits for the problem to resolve itself.
- Approach methods:
  - Predatory clinicians exist in the associated mental health fields and use grooming and seduction to overcome victim resistance and minimize chance of disclosure.
  - Many boundary-violating clinicians fall in love with a client, which causes them to risk their entire career.
  - Those using an approach-automatic pathway have a desire to act on their arousal but do not make active plans to offend; they respond to situational cues and passively allow circumstances to lead to a boundary violation.
- Choosing to engage in sexual contact with a client is far more complicated than a logical cost-analysis weighing the advantages and repercussions of the act. Influences on decision-making include:
  - biases and cognitive short cuts affect logical decision-making;
  - self-regulation ability can become depleted;
  - sexual arousal lowers inhibitions and impairs decision making (it also has a myopic effect, a form of tunnel vision in which the proximal goals of sexual gratification and pleasure temporarily override consideration about likely consequences); and
  - Cognitive distortions and faulty schemas, used to rationalize boundary violations.

- Interventions at this phase include:

  o seeking supervision and consultation;

  o actively considering the long-term consequences of the act rather than the more easily imagined short-term satisfaction it might bring; and

  o stopping seeing the client, even if temporarily.

References

Abbey, A. (1982). Sex differences in attributions for friendly behavior: Do males misperceive females' friendliness? *Journal of Personality and Social Psychology, 42*(5), 830.

Abel, G. G., Osborn, C. A., & Warberg, B. (1995). Cognitive-behavioral treatment for professional sexual misconduct. *Psychiatric Annals, 25*(2), 106–112.

Ariely, D., & Loewenstein, G. (2006). The heat of the moment: The effect of sexual arousal on sexual decision making. *Journal of Behavioral Decision Making, 19*(2), 87–98.

Bickley, J. A., & Beech, A. R. (2002). An investigation of the ward and hudson pathways model of the sexual offense process with child abusers. *Journal of Interpersonal Violence, 17*(4), 371–393.

Burns, D. D. (1989). *The feeling good handbook: Using the new mood therapy in everyday life.* New York: William Morrow & Co.

Carich, M. S., & Adkerson, D. L. (1995). *Adult sexual offender assessment packet.* Orwell, VT: Safer Society Press.

Craven, S., Brown, S., & Gilchrist, E. (2006). Sexual grooming of children: Review of literature and theoretical considerations. *Journal of Sexual Aggression, 12*(3), 287–299.

Farris, C., Treat, T. A., Viken, R. J., & McFall, R. M. (2008). Sexual coercion and the misperception of sexual intent. *Clinical Psychology Review, 28*(1), 48–66.

Finkelhor, D. (1984). *Child sexual abuse: New theory and research.* New York: Free Press, 1984.

Haidt, J. (2012). *The righteous mind: Why good people are divided by politics and religion.* New York: Vintage.

Jacques-Tiura, A. J., Abbey, A., Parkhill, M. R., & Zawacki, T. (2007). Why do some men misperceive women's sexual intentions more frequently than others do? An application of the confluence model. *Personality and Social Psychology Bulletin, 33*(11), 1467–1480.

Kahn, T. J. (1990). *Pathways: A guided workbook for youth beginning treatment.* Orwell, VT: Safer Society Press.

Lamb, D. H., Catanzaro, S. J., & Moorman, A. S. (2003). Psychologists reflect on their sexual relationships with clients, supervisees, and students: Occurrence, impact, rationales and collegial intervention. *Professional Psychology: Research and Practice, 34*(1), 102.

Luca, M., & and Boyden, M. (2014). "An elephant in the room: A grounded theory of experienced psychotherapists' reactions and attitudes to sexual attraction. In M. Luca (Ed.), *Sexual attraction in therapy: Clinical perspectives on moving beyond the taboo* (pp. 193–208). West Sussex, U K: John Wiley & Sons.

Martin, C., Godfrey, M., Meekums, B., & Madill, A. (2011). Managing boundaries under pressure: A qualitative study of therapists' experiences of sexual attraction in therapy. *Counselling and Psychotherapy Research, 11*(4), 248–256.

McNulty, N., Ogden, J., & Warren, F. (2013). 'Neutralizing the patient': Therapists' accounts of sexual boundary violations. *Clinical Psychology & Psychotherapy, 20*(3), 189–198.

Millar, B. M., Starks, T. J., Rendina, H. J., & Parsons, J. T. (2019). Three reasons to consider the role of tiredness in sexual risk-taking among gay and bisexual men. *Archives of Sexual Behavior, 48*(1), 383–395.

Millar, B. M., Starks, T. J., Rendina, H. J., & Parsons, J. T. (2019). Three reasons to consider the role of tiredness in sexual risk-taking among gay and bisexual men. *Archives of Sexual Behavior, 48*(1), 383–395.

Muraven, M., Tice, D. M., & Baumeister, R. F. (1998). Self-control as a limited resource: Regulatory depletion patterns. *Journal of Personality and Social Psychology, 74*(3), 774.

Palmer, C. A., & Alfano, C. A. (2017). Sleep and emotion regulation: An organizing, integrative review. *Sleep Medicine Reviews, 31*, 6–16.

Polaschek, D. L., & Ward, T. (2002). The implicit theories of potential rapists: What our questionnaires tell us. *Aggression and Violent Behavior, 7*(4), 385–406.

Sapolsky, R. M. (2017). *Behave: The biology of humans at our best and worst.* New York: Penguin.

Simon, H. A. (1979). Rational decision making in business organizations. *The American Economic Review, 69*(4), 493–513.

Skakoon-Sparling, S., Cramer, K. M., & Shuper, P. A. (2016). The impact of sexual arousal on elements of sexual decision making: Sexual self-restraint, motivational state, and self-control. *The Canadian Journal of Human Sexuality, 25*(2), 119–125.

Steele, C. M., & Josephs, R. A. (1990). Alcohol myopia: Its prized and dangerous effects. *American Psychologist, 45*(8), 921–933.

Tanner, J., & Brake, S. (2013). Exploring sex offender grooming [text file]. URL:www.kbsolutions.com/Grooming.pdf

van Dam, C. (2001). *Identifying child molesters: Preventing child sexual abuse by recognizing the patterns of the offenders.* Binghamton, NY: Haworth Maltreatment and Trauma Press/The Haworth Press, Inc.

Vohs, K. D., Baumeister, R. F., Schmeichel, B. J., Twenge, J. M., Nelson, N. M., & Tice, D. M. (2008). Making choices impairs subsequent self-control: A limited-resource account of decision making, self-regulation, and active initiative. *Journal of Personality and Social Psychology, 94*(5), 883–898.

Ward, T., & Hudson, S. M. (1998). A model of the relapse process in sexual offenders. *Journal of Interpersonal Violence, 13*, 700–725.

Ward, T., & Keenan, T. (1999). Child molesters' implicit theories. *Journal of Interpersonal Violence, 14*(8), 821–838.

Williams, R., Elliott, I. A., & Beech, A. R. (2013). Identifying sexual grooming themes used by internet sex offenders. *Deviant Behavior, 34*(2), 135–152.

Using Clients to Meet Unfulfilled Needs

6

Chapter 5 described the *choosing* phase of the Boundary Violation Cycle, the point at which a professional recognizes they are on a slippery slope, that sexual attraction is beginning to impact their ability to work with a client, and that risk of consequences is escalating. Logic dictates a clinician would make active efforts to avoid further progression along the cycle, but many choose instead to continue. That chapter explained that many factors influence this choice, including arousal, permissive self-talk, faulty underlying schemas, and depleted self-regulatory ability. This current chapter continues to build upon sexual decision-making by describing two models promulgating a belief that often-unconscious processing leads to poor sexual decisions; both find latent psychological forces compel a professional to continue on to a boundary violation. First, a psychodynamic conceptualization, one of the earliest and most enduring explanations for professional boundary violations, argues that such incidents are the end result of transference gone awry. The second explanatory model and one that is gaining increasing traction is the Good Lives Model, which proposes that individuals make counterproductive sexual decisions because they somehow fill an implicit but extremely important unmet need. Both of these will be explored in this chapter.

Let's return to our example of Jessica from earlier chapters, who recognize that her attraction to her patient Joseph has become both enthralling and worrisome. She must make a choice as to how to proceed: either avoid or approach (using terminology from Chapter 5). The psychodynamic perspective postulates that her attraction is a result of countertransference, an unconscious imprinting of Joseph with characteristics that have little to do with him but are more a reflection of her past unmet needs and experiences. The Good

Lives Model, in contrast, states that a romantic relationship with Joseph is a flawed effort to obtain an otherwise healthy prime human motivating factor: relatedness. Based on her dynamic risk factors (i.e., recent romantic separation, unsatisfying dating experiences, and the possible death of her mother), this makes perfect sense. Both conceptualizations state that these processes occur without conscious awareness. Choosing the right path when confronted with sexual arousal to a client is thus made even more complicated.

Sexual Boundary Violations Due to Transference

Infantile yearnings are revived and enacted in the context of therapy, often taking the form of sexualized dependent striving. When patients and/or therapists confuse these feelings with adult sexual wishes, the results may be disastrous. Unfortunately, this distinctions eludes too many people (Strasburger, Jorgenson, & Sutherland 1992, p. 545).

The earliest explanations for sexual boundary violations are based on psychodynamic conceptualizations, and they continue to predominate in the literature. Transference in a therapeutic relationship occurs when a client invests a treatment provider with qualities that are in reality a reflection of their unresolved and often-unconscious conflicts. Similarly, treatment professionals also project their own underlying vulnerabilities onto clients, which is called countertransference. During therapy both patient and client inevitably project their interpersonal issues onto one another (Hamilton & Spruill, 1999), which means that when attraction arises for the client, therapist, or both, this is in actuality a reflection of unconscious wishes and fears. A therapist, for example, is not the real target of a client's romantic and sexual attraction but is instead a temporary proxy until unconscious issues are resolved. Therapists must recognize that a patient's falling in love with them is the result of the dynamics of therapy and not due to providers' inherent charms (Freud, Strachey, Freud, & Richards, 1953).

Mismanaged transference can lead a client and professional to fall in love with each other, though Celenza (2017) questions whether love occurring in the dynamics of therapy is equivalent to love in other romantic but non-professional relationships. In her 2007 book *Sexual Boundary Violations*, she questions, "What are the circumstances under which two adults may be considered consenting, relatively free of transference-based pressures and structured power imbalances?" (p. 65). Relationships between a mental health professional and a client certainly do not reflect these circumstances. The therapist, aware that they are falling in love, avoids clinical consultation with a peer or supervisor because they are afraid of losing the patient (Simon, 1991). A patient may also demonstrate signs of improvement arising from the change of tone in the clinical relationship; Simon (1991), one of the most prolific researchers on the topic, found patients often report temporary improvement in symptoms when a therapeutic relationship devolves into a love affair. These early and superficial improvements do not negate the recognized constellation of short- and long-term psychological harms that follow. A love relationship also interferes with clinical judgment and leads to failure to properly treat a patient.

In their introduction to a 2017 edition of *Psychoanalytic Psychology* dedicated to the topic of sexual boundary violations, Steinberg and Alpert (2017) highlight the links between countertransference and sexual boundary violations, particularly noting the role of erotic transference. Book (1995) refers to erotic transference as reverential, sensual, or sexual feelings toward the therapist arising from unresolved developmental issues. Ladson and Welton (2007) differentiate between erotic transference, which consists of positive feelings towards a professional accompanied by sexual fantasies that the patient understands to be unrealistic, and eroticized transference that consists of irrational sexual preoccupation with the professional. Both forms of transference are very difficult for clinicians to manage, who either tend to become aloof in an effort to maintain emotional distance or become inappropriately involved with a client. Gabbard (1994) determined erotic transference is one of the most powerful and challenging phenomena in therapy and that it can interfere with a professional's ability to maintain a dual state of awareness in which he or she is both a participant and observer of the treatment experience.

Simon (1995) posits that professionals struggling with crises, transitions, and even disappointments may consciously or unconsciously use a patient's sexualized transference as a means of bolstering their damaged ego, a concept he called narcissistic repair.

In sum, the psychodynamic conceptualization of sexual boundary violations states they are a result of unconscious dynamics, particularly transference, occurring in the confines of the therapeutic relationship, which already fosters intimacy as part of its process. Without supervision, clinical consultation, reflection, and possibly therapy for the clinician, these dynamics can perniciously escalate to boundary crossings and an eventual violation. Simon (1989) states,

> [I]t would be naïve to underestimate the power of transference and countertransference feelings. It can be extraordinarily difficult for the therapist and patient in the throes of such feelings to assess the dangers

of their situation. While the therapist may intellectually know that treatment boundaries are being crossed, powerful countertransference feelings may weaken the will to resist.

(p. 107)

Inappropriate management of transference was cited in one of the first successful legal cases brought against a clinician (*Zipkin v Freeman* in 1968), and Hamilton and Spruill (1999) decry that clinical supervision has moved away from discussing transference and countertransference issues, which leaves many practitioners unprepared for the erotic attraction towards or from a client or mutuality of this feeling.

Sexual Boundary Violations Due to Unmet Needs

The first 2000 edition of *American Psychologist* was dedicated to the then nascent practice of positive psychology, which lead authors Seligman and Csikszentmihalyi (2000) described as "a change in the focus of psychology from preoccupation only with repairing the worst things in life to also building positive qualities" (p. 5). No longer, the authors championed, should psychology focus only on adversity, trauma, mental illness, and healing; instead it should give similar credence to assisting people to thrive, flourish, and develop their capacities to live meaningful and fulfilling lives.

Positive psychology has continued to mature and develop since the release of this first seminal work, and subjects subsumed now include optimism, happiness, love, gratitude, forgiveness, positive relationships, and healthy institutions. Seligman's (2012) PERMA model offers a synthesis of research in the field and states that five core elements comprise the necessary ingredients for a satisfying life. PERMA is an acronym standing for:

- **Positive emotions and feeling good** – This includes cultivating optimism and judiciously maximizing the number of positive emotions one experiences, particularly those arising from intellectual stimulation and creativity in contrast to pleasure, which is a result of satiating bodily needs, such as hunger and thirst.
- **Engagement** – Participating in activities that completely absorb one in the moment, a state also commonly referred to as "flow" (Csikszentmihalyi, 1997).
- **Relationships** – One of the strongest predictors of a satisfying life is engagement in meaningful relationships.

- **Meaning** – Determining one's purpose in life and living in a way that brings it to fruition.
- **Accomplishments** – Setting realistic goals – both short- and long-term – and making efforts to accomplish them.

Developments in the field of positive psychology indicate that incorporating PERMA into one's life leads to a richer, more meaningful, and satisfying life.

Strengths and Values

One of the cornerstones of the Meaning component of PERMA is character strengths. Seligman (2012) identified 24 characters strengths aggregated into six categories:

- **love:** intimacy, kindness, sociability;
- **wisdom and knowledge:** creativity, judgment, curiosity, love of learning, perspective;
- **courage:** bravery, perseverance, integrity, enthusiasm;
- **justice:** sense of responsibility, fairness, leadership;
- **temperance:** forgiveness, humility, caution, self-control; and
- **transcendence:** appreciation, gratitude, optimism, humor, spirituality.

Positive psychology urges individuals to identify their character strengths and use them frequently. We do not have all of the above strengths and we obtain more satisfaction from some over others. People seeking out situations in which to use their identified strengths report more life satisfaction. Peterson and Seligman's (2004) conceptualization of character strengths evolved through cross-cultural research into virtues that occur across the globe and have been present throughout history.

Similar to character strengths, Lineham (2015), in her formation of dialectical behavior therapy (DBT), notes the importance of core values. Part of treatment consists of helping individuals identify their personal core values and assisting them to act upon them in their day-to-day lives. Her values include:

- attending to relationships;
- being part of a group;
- being powerful and influencing others;
- achieving things in life;

- living a life of pleasure and satisfaction;
- keeping life full of exciting events, relationships, and things;
- behaving respectfully;
- being self-directed;
- being a spiritual person;
- achieving security;
- recognizing the universal of all things;
- contributing to the larger community;
- working on self-development; and
- having integrity.

Acceptance and Commitment Therapy (ACT), a relatively new paradigm in mental health treatment, also recognizes the concept of underlying values; Harris (2009) uses a metaphor of a compass, in that values offer a direction as to how a person can lead a meaningful life. ACT assists clients to identify their values and develop a values-congruent life. Some core values noted in ACT include:

- spirituality;
- leisure;
- personal growth;
- health;
- community and environment;
- family relationships;
- intimate relationships; and
- social relationships.

In sum, living a values-congruent life, or, using positive psychology terminology, maximizing use of one's character strengths, has been found to lead to a more satisfying life. When people are unable to live by their values, depression, dissatisfaction, and existential crises can result. Can this also however lead to poor sexual decision-making? The Good Lives Model, which will be addressed next, proposes it indeed can.

The Good Lives Model

The Good Lives Model was developed to address obvious limitations to the then and still current risk management approach to working with convicted sex offenders. This latter approach focuses on avoidance of further harm in the community rather than improving the quality of offenders' lives, which may lead better outcomes. Ward and Gannon (2006) identified risk management as necessary but not sufficient for successful treatment. The Good Lives Model is a strengths-based approach that enhances offenders' capabilities in attaining *primary human goods*. According to Ward and Gannon (2006), primary goods "are states of affairs, states of mind, personal characteristics, activities, or experiences that are sought for their own sake and are likely to increase psychological well-being if achieved" (p. 79). Similarly, Ward, Mann, and Gannon (2007) determined that people are likely to be more satisfied with their lives if they have access to the various types of primary human goods. Also, each person gives more weight or priority to some goods over others. These conclusions are very much in accordance with the character strengths and core values described earlier. The primary goal of treatment using the Good Lives Model is to install in offenders the knowledge, skills, and competencies to gain primary human goods in an acceptable manner. The primary human goods identified are:

- life (including healthy living and functioning);
- knowledge (how well informed one feels about things that are important to them);
- excellence in play (hobbies and recreational pursuits);
- excellence in work (including mastery experiences);
- excellence in agency (autonomy, power and self-directedness);
- inner peace (freedom from emotional turmoil and stress);
- relatedness (including intimate, romantic, and familial relationships);
- community (connection to wider social groups);
- spirituality (in the broad sense of finding meaning and purpose in life);
- pleasure (feeling good in the here and now); and
- creativity (expressing oneself through alternative forms)

Andrews, Bonta, and Wormith (2011) summarized several core principles of the Good Lives Model, including:

- human behavior at its highest level is intrinsically motivated;
- behavior reflects genetic predispositions in combination with personal narratives and identities associated with the pursuit of aspirations;
- internal and/or external conditions interfere with the achievement of human goods; and
- people engage in crime because they lack the capabilities to realize valued outcomes in personally fulfilling and socially acceptable ways.

Willis, Yates, Gannon, and Ward (2013) propose that primary goods are met through instrumental means (also known as secondary goods), and they give examples of a primary good of knowledge being met through attending university and the primary good of community being met through belonging to a sports group. Secondary goods are the activities individuals undertake in pursuit of primary human goods and the attainment of their life goals. These secondary routes to achieving one's primary goods are where problems arise; individuals often use maladaptive and flawed methods to achieve their primary goods. Primary human goods by themselves are not problematic. Lindsay, Ward, Morgan, and Wilson (2007) stress that unattained primary goods may remain obfuscated from conscious awareness; individuals engage in instrumental acts such as sex, which on the surface appears to be motivated purely by arousal, attraction, or romance, that might in actuality be efforts to attain a primary human good. Sex offending against children for example may be a consequence of an effort to attain a primary good of relatedness. For others, the primary good of establishing a sense of agency or autonomy is obtained via sexual aggression. Mental health professionals whose primary human goods are unsatisfied might use a sexual or romantic relationship with a client as a secondary route to obtaining gratification all the while lacking recognition that this is a motivating force for their behavior.

Ward and Gannon (2006) differentiate between direct and indirect sexual routes for attainment of primary goods. Those who use the direct route have developed a habitual means of obtaining primary human goods in the form of sexual activity. This path would be typical of predatory clinicians. In contrast those on the indirect route, which would subsume the majority of professionals engaging in boundary violations, find their pursuit of a good or set of goods frustrated and unachieved thus resulting in dissatisfaction. This results in a "ripple effect" (p. 86), leading to unanticipated effects; a chain-of-events emanating from an unfulfilled primary good leads to maladaptive efforts to attain it, which, as is the topic of this text, could be sexual activity with a client. Unfulfilled primary goods leave a person vulnerable to changing circumstances.

According to Yates, Prescott, and Ward (2010) a preventative effort using the Good Lives Model would include:

- education about primary human goods and the use of secondary means to attain them, including inappropriate and harmful approaches;
- increasing the scope of one's primary goods when a person narrowly focuses on a very few thus precluding the achievement of other goods. All are important in a satisfying life although some are always idiosyncratically valued over others;

- recognizing conflict between primary goods. As an example, a goal of autonomy often conflicts with a goal of relatedness. A preventative method would help a person recognize these implicit contrasts and conflicts and develop a plan for exploring and resolving contradictions; and
- equipping individuals with the capabilities and resources to obtain their goals in socially acceptable ways.

Conclusions

This chapter expounded on the difficulties professionals face when experiencing sexual attraction to a client. What appears to be an easy choice – moving away from a sexual boundary violation – can be exceedingly difficult. Already cudgeled by the impact of arousal and permissive cognitive distortions and schemas, we find that there are also underlying forces, of which we may be completely unaware or only partially cognizant of, that are driving behavior. The psychodynamic perspective informs us that transference and countertransference, particularly the dynamic of falling in love with a client, make professional consultation, the recommended option, unlikely to occur. Not only is a professional embarrassed by this occurrence, but disclosure to a supervisor or colleague risks that possibility that they will be told the relationship must end. Who wants to lose somebody they love? The Good Lives Model – built upon decades of research into the influence of goals, aspirations, and self-actualization as motivators for behaviors – finds that clinicians who are unable to satisfy their own idiosyncratic Good Lives Model may make maladaptive attempts to attain it in the clinical realm.

These two models are not mutually exclusive; countertransference issues and unattained good life priorities can play out simultaneously. As is a core theme through this book, these processes are not static. A clinician may capably manage transference and countertransference until unexpected life changes make him more vulnerable. An unattained primary good may perniciously haunt a person's life though never lead to more than vague satisfaction. However, a specific patient, life transition or crisis, or employment in an environment in which clinical boundaries are frequently elided can lead a festering dissatisfaction to devolve into active use of a client to attain this good. Both of these processes often manifest without conscious awareness that they are even occurring

The last two chapters have shown that there are numerous forces at play when intrusive sexual attraction occurs in a clinical setting. Quickly it becomes a slippery slope on which one will not be able to regain balance if left unaddressed too long. To paraphrase a cautionary note by Simon (1989), the forces described in these chapters weaken the will to resist moving away from a boundary violation and instead perniciously compel one to advance towards it.

Summary

- Two current models – the psychodynamic perspective and the Good Lives Model – conclude unconscious and latent psychological forces influence sexual decision-making.
- Psychodynamic theorizing about professional boundary violations is predominant in the literature. It surmises that mismanaged transference and countertransference are the root causes of boundary violations.
- Transference in a therapeutic relationship occurs when a client invests a treatment provider with qualities that are in reality a reflection of their unresolved and often-unconscious conflicts. Similarly, treatment professionals also project their own underlying vulnerabilities onto clients, which is called countertransference.
- Transference is often difficult for clinicians to manage, and they tend to become aloof in an effort to maintain emotional distance or become inappropriately involved with a client.
- Mismanaged transference can lead a client and professional to fall in love with each other.
- The Good Lives Model builds upon decades of research into the influence of goals, aspirations, and self-actualization as motivators for behaviors.
- Individuals engage in instrumental acts such as sex, which on the surface appear to be motivated purely by arousal, attraction, or romance, that might in actuality be an effort to attain a primary human good.
- The primary goal of treatment using the Good Lives Model is to install in individuals the knowledge, skills, and competencies to gain primary human goods in an acceptable manner.
- These two models are not mutually exclusive; countertransference issues and unattained good life priorities can play out simultaneously.

References

Andrews, D. A., Bonta, J., & Wormith, J. S. (2011). The risk-need-responsivity (RNR) model: Does adding the Good Lives Model contribute to effective crime prevention? *Criminal Justice and Behavior, 38*(7), 735–755.

Book, H. E. (1995). The "erotic transference": Some technical and countertransferential difficulties. *American Journal of Psychotherapy, 49*(4), 504–513.

Celenza, A. (2007). *Sexual boundary violations.* Lanham, MD: Jason Aronson.

Celenza, A. (2017). Lessons on or about the couch: What sexual boundary transgressions can teach us about everyday practice. *Psychoanalytic Psychology, 34*(2), 157.

Csikszentmihalyi, M. (1997). *Finding flow: The psychology of engagement with everyday life.* New York: Basic Books.

Freud, S., Strachey, J., Freud, A., & Richards, A. (1953). *The standard edition of the complete psychological works of sigmund freud: Tr. from the German.* London, United Kingdom: Hogarth Press.

Gabbard, G. O. (1994). On love and lust in erotic transference. *Journal of the American Psychoanalytic Association, 42*(2), 385–386.

Hamilton, J. C., & Spruill, J. (1999). Identifying and reducing risk factors related to trainee–Client sexual misconduct. *Professional Psychology: Research and Practice, 30*(3), 318.

Harris, R. (2009). *ACT made simple: An easy-to-read primer on acceptance and commitment therapy.* Oakland, CA: New Harbinger Publications.

Ladson, D., & Welton, R. (2007). Recognizing and managing erotic and eroticized transferences. *Psychiatry (Edgmont), 4*(4), 47–50.

Lindsay, W. R., Ward, T., Morgan, T., & Wilson, I. (2007). Self-regulation of sex offending, future pathways and the Good Lives Model: Applications and problems. *Journal of Sexual Aggression, 13*(1), 37–50.

Lineham, M.M. (2015). *DBT skills training manual, second edition.* New York: Guilford.

Peterson, C., & Seligman, M. E. P. (2004). *Character strengths and virtues: A classification and handbook.* New York: Oxford University Press/Washington,DC: American Psychological Association.

Seligman, M. E. (2012). *Flourish: A visionary new understanding of happiness and well-being.* New York: Simon and Schuster.

Seligman, M. E., & Csikszentmihalyi, M. (2000). Positive psychology: An introduction. *American Psychologist, 55*(1), 5–14.

Simon, R. I. (1989). Sexual exploitation of patients: How it begins before it happens. *Psychiatric Annals, 19*(2), 104–112.

Simon, R. I. (1991). Psychological injury caused by boundary violation precursors to therapist-patient sex. *Psychiatric Annals, 21*(10), 614–619.

Simon, R. I. (1995). The natural history of therapist sexual misconduct: Identification and prevention. *Psychiatric Annals, 25*(2), 90–94.

Steinberg, A. L., & Alpert, J. L. (2017). Sexual boundary violations: An agenda demanding more consideration. *Psychoanalytic Psychology, 34*(2), 221.

Strasburger, L. H., Jorgenson, L., & Sutherland, P. (1992). The prevention of psychotherapist sexual misconduct: Avoiding the slippery slope. *American Journal of Psychotherapy, 46*(4), 544–555.

Ward, T., & Gannon, T. A. (2006). Rehabilitation, etiology, and self-regulation: The comprehensive Good Lives Model of treatment for sexual offenders. *Aggression and Violent Behavior, 11*(1), 77–94.

Ward, T., Mann, R. E., & Gannon, T. A. (2007). The Good Lives Model of offender rehabilitation: Clinical implications. *Aggression and Violent Behavior, 12*(1), 87–107.

Willis, G. M., Yates, P. M., Gannon, T. A., & Ward, T. (2013). How to integrate the Good lives model into treatment programs for sexual offending: An introduction and overview. *Sexual Abuse, 25*(2), 123–142.

Yates, P. M., Prescott, D., & Ward, T. (2010). *Applying the Good Lives and self-regulation models to sex offender treatment.* Brandon, VT: Safer Society.

Non-Sexual
Boundary Crossings

7

[T]he road to sexual misconduct is strewn with boundary violations ...
(Simon 1995, p. 92)

Attraction between a client and a therapist is common and can be beneficial for the treatment process simply because we tend to work better with people we genuinely like. Ladany et al. (1997) for example found therapists reported they were more invested, caring, and attentive when attracted to a client. Similarly, Giovazolias and Davis (2001) interviewed counseling psychologists about their experiences of sexual attraction to clients; they reported becoming more interested in clients' problems and that these feelings enhanced their therapeutic work with the clients. Conversely, consider the work on implicit bias, which are attitudes or stereotypes about groups that perniciously affect our understanding, actions, and decisions in an unconscious manner. In the clinical realm they have been shown to lead to increased blinking, speech errors, decreased smiling, decreased eye contact, a tendency to impulsively move away from targets of bias, and to sit a greater distance during sessions (Boysen, 2010). In contrast, when we find ourselves attracted to a person we engage in the opposite behaviors, such as more smiling and sitting closer. The purpose of the latter behaviors is not to manipulate a client – there is no hidden agenda for future sexual or romantic involvement – it is simply a human characteristic to treat those we find attractive in a warmer and friendlier manner. However, when attraction leads to boundary crossings, problems can accrue, often very quickly, and with limited awareness they are occurring.

"What am I doing?" Jessica asks herself frequently regarding her work with Joseph. Her initial and seemingly innocuous self-disclosures to this patient have become even more revealing. She has now disclosed the neighborhood in which she lives, the fact that she co-habits with female roommates, and some of the frustrations she has with her job. Sessions are becoming more social and less clinical. Joseph is now in the habit of quickly hugging her at the end of their session.

Jessica acknowledges she should, at the least, talk to a colleague about these boundary crossings. She doesn't though because she is embarrassed, confident in her ability to manage her emotions and behavior, and doesn't want to risk the possibility that she will be directed to end or at least change the dynamics of sessions with Joseph.

With these considerations in mind she is still unprepared as to how to respond when Joseph, sheepishly and with great hesitation, asks if she is currently dating anybody.

Crossings and Violations

Gutheil and Gabbard's (1993) highly influential work on clinical boundaries differentiated between boundary crossings and boundary violations and continues to be used as a guide in clinical decision-making. According to Smith and Fitzpatrick (1995),

> Boundary crossing is a nonpejorative term that describes departures from commonly accepted clinical practice that may or may not benefit the client … A boundary violation, on the other hand, is a departure from accepted practice that places the client or the therapeutic process at serious risk.
>
> (p. 500)

Sawyer and Prescott (2011) further elaborate upon these conceptualizations by stating that crossings and violations range along a continuum, extending from acts having less potential to harm a client, to those with significant risk of harm. This conclusion echoes the earlier work of Gutheil and Gabbard (1993), who emphasized that crossing boundaries "may at times be salutary, at times neutral, and at times harmful" and that the nature, clinical usefulness, and impact of a particular crossing "can only be assessed by a careful attention to the clinical context" (pp. 188–189).

Every mental health association recognizes sexual contact with a client is a boundary violation. Such violations are almost always preceded by a series of boundary crossings that become increasingly intrusive and detrimental to the client's welfare. When though does a boundary crossing go from being "salutary" to "neutral" to "harmful?" For example, when does clinician self-disclosure, the most recognized boundary crossing preceding sexual contact between clinician and patient, transition from therapeutic to malfeasance? When does extending a session transform from concern about a critical issue to manipulation? A predatory clinician using gradually progressing boundary crossings as a means of grooming and seduction most certainly is worthy of condemnation. A lovesick clinician hesitatingly testing boundaries to monitor whether a patient feels the same way might appear less overtly objectionable but is still objectively inappropriate. In short, any boundary-crossing behavior a clinician recognizes as advancing him or her closer to a sexual boundary violation is contrary to the therapeutic process. Smith and Fitzpatrick (1995), in their review of boundary guidelines in psychotherapy, offer three principles that help determine whether a crossing is appropriate or inappropriate. First is *abstinence*, in which therapists refrain from seeking personal gratification other than that which is derived from being a part of the therapeutic process. The second, *neutrality*, states the client's agenda is the primary consideration in therapy. Finally, mental health professionals should strive to enhance a client's *autonomy and independence* and not engage in activities that would otherwise restrict these qualities. Sawyer and Prescott (2011) summarize the above by stating,

> Clear boundaries protect the client from harm, ensure that the client interests are paramount, and promote the objectivity and neutrality of the professional. Boundary violations put the objectivity or neutrality of the professional at risk or creates a conflict of interest.
>
> (p. 372)

Pope and Keith-Spiegel (2008) remind us, "No shortcuts in logic can free us from the responsibility of thinking through the nature and implications of what we are doing with our clients" (p. 644). The unpredictable outcome of a boundary crossing is affected by a client's history, symptoms, and diagnosis; a professional's theoretical orientation (e.g., humanistic therapists have different beliefs about the appropriateness of boundary crossings in comparison to those utilizing a psychodynamic approach); and the immediate circumstances.

Types of Boundary Crossings & Violations

Sexual boundary violations are preceded by behaviors and interactions that in the beginning appear to have nothing to do with sex (Tschan, 2014). In their study of client victims, Somer and Saadon (1999) found a process of gradual boundary violation characterized by therapist disclosure; therapists began to reveal feelings, emotions, and information related to their personal lives. Some talked about their preferred foods, films, or poetry, while others talked about their emotional, marital, or sexual problems. Some disclosed to the patients how "special" they were to them.

Researchers have retrospectively examined self-reports of transgressing professionals and their victims and compiled a list of common non-sexual boundary crossings preceding a sexual boundary violation (e.g. Simon, 1991). The following have been noted in the literature:

- self-disclosure;
- scheduling a client as the last patient of the day;
- sessions become more frequent;
- sessions become increasingly more social and less clinical;
- asking unnecessary sexual questions;
- touching of patient, including hugs and embraces;
- kissing;
- having excessive contact with the patient, including telephone, social media, texting, etc.;
- patient becomes a confidant;
- neutrality of professional slowly erodes;
- becoming lax with fees or stops billing;
- exchanging gifts;
- lending money to a client;
- going to a client's special events (such as a graduation or funeral);
- going to a social gathering knowing in advance a client will be present;
- asking the patient to engage to perform household or office tasks; and
- meetings for lunch or dinner.

Several researchers have aggregated the above list into a smaller number of descriptive categories. For example, Smith and Fitzpatrick (1995) formulated four broad categories of boundary concerns:

- First, *dual relationships,* a common ethical concern and defined by Gottlieb (1993) in his landmark article on the topic as occurring when a professional maintains a simultaneous personal relationship with a client such as friend, family member, student or business partner.
- Second, *non-erotic physical contact* (e.g., a reassuring touch or hug), which Smith and Fitzpatrick recognize could be an appropriate response at

certain times or with certain clients, but that nonetheless could lead to unforeseen consequences. Pope, Tabachnick, and Keith-Spiegel (1987) surveyed psychologists and found that handshakes with clients were widely practiced and considered ethical, hugging occurred far less commonly but was still considered ethical, and that kissing was practiced with the lowest frequency and was considered ethical only under rare circumstances.

- *Self-disclosure*, the third category, can be beneficial when used for the client's benefit within the context of the therapeutic process. However, as has already been stated, it is also the seeming gateway boundary crossing progressing towards a sexual violation. Self-disclosure has been and continues to remain one of the most contentious topics in the mental health fields.
- *Therapist-client sexual contact*, the final category, is described as the most disruptive and damaging boundary violation.

In a similar effort, but for much more sexually specific behaviors, Stake and Oliver (1991), interviewed licensed psychologists about their definitions of professional sexual misconduct. Factor analysis of the responses led to the formulation of three patterns: First, *overt sexual behavior* was denoted by kissing, exposure, fondling of genital areas, oral sex, and intercourse. The second pattern *touching behavior* was seen in examples of touching the face, hair, or neck; hugging; or holding hands with clients. Finally, *suggestive behavior* was exemplified by sexual humor and suggestive looks or remarks.

As stated earlier, boundary crossings are not necessarily harmful and, on some occasions, can facilitate treatment. Pope (1994) for example decried a growing specter of "touch anxiety" in the mental health field in which non-sexual human touch in a clinical setting is seen as inherently dangerous, wrong, harmful, and risking legal repercussions. He does offer several qualifications though, particularly physical contact being incompatible with some theoretical orientations and that for some clients physical touch is unwanted, intrusive, or even frightening. Still, the above boundary crossings, even when they do not lead to sexual engagement, can nonetheless compromise treatment. It is always the professional's responsibility to maintain boundaries. Many patients enter treatment unaware of appropriate boundaries in therapy, with histories of boundary violations, including sexual abuse, and/or presenting with chronic boundary issues symptomatic of underlying psychopathology.

The Abstinence Violation Effect and Entrapment

Self-deception allows one to cross boundaries of growing intimacy. As has been indicated throughout this book, sexual-decision making can be complicated and is influenced by numerous factors, including arousal, distorted self-talk, countertransference, unmet primary human goods, and the current circumstances in one's life. Thus, professionals convince themselves to continue on their current course in spite of known consequences; recall that Lamb, Catanzaro, and Moorman (2003), in their survey of practicing psychologists who had engaged in prohibited sexual relationships with clients, supervisees, and students, found that 28% of responses indicated continuation of the behavior even after recognizing it was problematic and/or unethical.

Even when a professional recognizes that boundary crossings are occurring it is often difficult to stop. This is explained by the principles of the Abstinence Violation Effect (AVE) and entrapment. The AVE, a concept borrowed from literature on substance abuse states that the breaking of a self-imposed rule tends to lead one to continue on a current course of action (Marlatt & Gordon, 1985). A person in recovery from intoxicating substances who engages in a subsequent singular use episode experiences cognitive (e.g., "I'll never be able to stop using.") and affective (e.g., hopelessness; shame) responses leading to a complete relapse. In other word, a "lapse" or single-use episode has the potential to progress to a full-blown relapse. We have all experienced the AVE in our lives. How many people have promised to eat only a handful of potato chips and soon found themselves devouring the entire bag? Another common example is gym or health club attendance; promises to work out three times a week are much easier to elide once we have skipped a day or two of the activity. According to the principles of the AVE, once a self-imposed promise regarding behavior has been broken, individuals can more easily continue on a path contrary to these promises.

The AVE has been incorporated into work with sex offenders as a relapse prevention tool (e.g., Wheeler, George, & Marlatt, 2006). Offenders can either recognize they are engaging in a risky behavior and stop or, after feeling guilt and hopelessness about their perceived inability to change, continue onto the next phase of their cycle. Mental health professionals, during the course of the non-sexual boundary crossings, have innumerable reflection points: the first intimate self-disclosure; the first extra-office non-clinical contact; and the first disclosure of romantic or sexual attraction. At each of these junctures clinicians experience competing forces, one compelling them to advance to intimate contact while another urging them to resist due to the dangers that each one of these intensifying behaviors portends. Self-imposed promises to stop after self-disclosure, texting, or social engagements can be broken one after another, leading a clinician to feel powerless to stop the process.

The AVE is further compounded by *entrapment* (also referred to as the sunk cost fallacy), described by Brockner et al. (1982) as situations in which "decision-makers feel compelled to continue investing their resources in order to justify previous costs incurred in the pursuit of some goal" (p. 248). Individuals become entrapped when they continue to invest in an unfavorable situation rather than ending it due to resources previously invested such as time, money, and effort. Katz, Tirone, and Schukrafft (2012), for example, found that women in abusive and violent relationships are more likely to remain with a partner when they had already invested significant time and resources. Clinicians engaging in boundary crossings recognize they may have already transgressed ethical obligations and put their reputation and career in jeopardy; the entrapment principle suggests this investment would lead them to continue on their path.

The AVE and entrapment are facilitated by cognitive distortions. Pope and Keith-Spiegel (2008) identified several common cognitive distortions that can lead to professional boundary crossings:

- What happens outside the psychotherapy session has nothing to do with therapy itself.
- Crossing a boundary with a therapy client has the same meaning as doing the same thing with someone who is not a client.
- Our understanding of a boundary crossing is also the client's understanding of the boundary crossing.
- A boundary crossing that is therapeutic for one client will also be therapeutic for another client.
- If we ourselves do not see any self-interest, problems, conflicts of interest, unintended consequences, major risks, or potential downsides to crossing a particular boundary, then there aren't any.
- Self-disclosure is always therapeutic because it shows authenticity, transparency, and trust.

Self-Assessment, Consultation, and Supervision

Early recognition of boundary crossings is essential since the AVE and entrapment make it increasingly difficult to reign in one's behavior. Plaut (2008) urges that professionals engage in ongoing "progressive boundary analysis", in which they consider the consequences of boundary crossings. However, self-deception makes this a fault-laden task necessitating reliance on more objective forms of introspection and reflection, typically self-assessment, consultation, and supervision.

Self-Assessment

Simon (1995) suggested that clinicians engage in "spot checks" to evaluate the possibility of boundary crossings in clinical interactions by asking themselves two questions. First, is an intervention for the benefit of the therapist or for the sake of the patient's treatment? Second, is the treatment intervention part of a series of boundary crossings? Pope and Keith-Spiegel (2008) directs professionals to pay attention to uneasy feelings or doubts regarding an intervention that might be perceived as a boundary crossing; many transgressors ignore or minimize the significance of these sensations. Also, they recommend imagining the best and worst outcomes that could occur following a crossing. Finally, they urge clinicians to be familiar with professional guidelines, ethics codes, legislation, and case law as they apply to crossings.

Hamilton and Spruill (1999) developed a comprehensive checklist that clinicians can use to reflect on likely and common boundary crossings. Considerations include:

- Do you find it difficult to set limits on the demands your client makes of you?
- Do you accept phone calls from your client at home or your office when the client needs you to: (a) help with a "crisis;" (b) deal with minor problems; or (c) alleviate his or her loneliness or meet his or her need to talk to someone who "understands?"
- Do you make statements such as "This is not my usual practice; I ordinarily don't do this, but, in your case ..." or "Under the circumstances, it seems OK to ..."?
- Do you find yourself wanting to rescue your client from some situation or behavior that is detrimental to them?
- Do you find yourself talking about your client to others?
- Does your client occupy your thoughts outside office hours?
- Do you hope you will "run into" your client at the grocery store, social settings, and so forth?
- Is it becoming progressively easier and more satisfying to share intimate details of your own life with your client?
- Do you find opportunities to talk about non-therapy issues with your client?

- Do you take care to dress or look more attractive than usual for a particular client?
- Do you find yourself wondering what the client thinks about you?
- Do you make excuses to talk with your client by phone?
- Do you find yourself looking forward to seeing a particular client (or type of client) and feeling disappointed if they cancel the session?
- Do you regularly extend the session for one client but not for others?
- Do you regularly start the session early, end it late, or both for one client?
- Do you schedule a particular client at times that afford the opportunity to linger, or to walk out of the clinic together, and so forth?
- Do you schedule the client after regular office hours because your schedule or the client's schedule does not permit regular office hours?
- Have you offered to do such things as give the client a ride home, give tutoring in a difficult class, or arrange a meeting outside the therapy hour or place?
- Are you concerned about the client's feelings toward you, or your feelings toward the client?

Epstein and Simon (1990) developed the Exploitation Index, a self-assessment questionnaire for therapists to identify early warning indicators of boundary violations in a therapeutic relationship. It is comprised of seven subscales:

1. generalized boundary violations;
2. eroticism;
3. dependency;
4. exhibitionism;
5. power seeking;
6. greediness; and
7. enabling.

Responses to the given questions range from "never" to "often." Sample questions include:

- Do you feel a sense of excitement or longing when you think of a patient or anticipate her/his visit?
- Do you touch your patients (exclude handshake)?
- Do you seek social contact with patients outside of clinically scheduled visits?

Epstein, Simon, and Kay (1992) later evaluated the usefulness of the Exploitation Index in a survey of 532 psychiatrists; 43% reported that at least one item alerted them to behavior they thought could have been counterproductive to treatment and 29% found that they were stimulated to make specific changes in future treatment practice.

Consultation and Supervision

Using colleagues or clinical supervision to identify boundary crossings is the most consistent recommendation in the literature. However, we know that the topic is also frequently elided in these settings. Above-mentioned Hamilton and Spruill (1999) suggest that any topics that a clinician would be embarrassed or uncomfortable to discuss with a colleague or supervisor are most certainly the topics that *need* to be discussed in these venues. They devised the following five questions, which are specific to supervision and consultation; affirmative answers suggest that significant boundary crossings are occurring or are on the verge of transpiring:

- Do you find yourself getting defensive about particular clients or certain issues (e.g., you bristle when a supervisor suggests that there is non-progress being made and a referral is in order)?
- Are you reluctant to talk about transference or boundary issues, particularly feelings related to sexual attraction by or to the client?
- Do you find it difficult to tell your treatment team or supervisor some details related to your client?
- Is there anything that you "try not to talk about" concerning a particular client?
- Do you find yourself putting off seeking supervision or consultation about a particular client or issue?

The goal of self-assessment, consultation, and supervision is corrective action. The professional stops engaging in boundary crossings and judiciously changes course in the therapy process with the indicated client before an irrevocable boundary violation occurs.

Coping with a Client's Attraction

It is not uncommon for a client to express their attraction to their treatment provider, and whether the feeling is mutual or not the same process of self-monitoring and supervision/consultation remains the recommended approach. How though does one manage the sexual and/or romantic attraction of a client? Luca and Boyden (2014), through interviews with practicing psychotherapists, found that fear of hurting a client's feelings led many to ignore the issue and hope that it would dissipate, a style labeled in this text as avoidant-passive. Others became defensive and engaged in authoritative, firm, intellectualizing, and disengaging behaviors. Some simply found a reason to terminate treatment. Instead, the authors suggest we handle it as we would any other emotions in session, such as anger, through use of a non-shaming and exploratory approach. Just as professionals can grow from processing their arousal, so too can clients. Goodyear and Shumate (1996) offer an example of a client learning he can have a strong feeling for another person and still not act on them. In the words of Luca and Boyden, "Clients' therapy will only go so far as the therapist is able to travel. Examine your attitudes to client sexual attraction as these will impact on the level of depth you are psychologically prepared to delve into" (2014, p. 205). Again, supervision or consultation should be concurrent.

Others remind us that the feelings of elation that often follow upon learning about a client's attraction should quickly be tempered with the realization that we are dealing with transference. As stated earlier, therapists must understand that a patient's falling in love with them is the result of the dynamics of therapy and not the providers' inherent charms (Freud, Strachey, Freud, & Richards, 1953). Students and practitioners generally new to the field, lacking extensive therapy experience, may be particularly prone to misinterpret the true source of a client's feelings and believe attraction is based on personal attributes rather than professional role (Hamilton & Spruill, 1999).

A recurrent argument in the field is whether it is ever appropriate to self-disclose one's attraction to a client. In an early study, Pope et al. (1987) found most psychologists reported it was unethical and likely harmful to disclose erotic feelings to clients, and this continues to be the majority opinion in spite of the frequently cited article by Giovazolias and Davis (2001), which found that the therapists who chose to disclose their feelings found their attraction benefitted therapy, compared with the therapists who did not disclose. Bridges (1998) concluded that clinician self-disclosure of attraction was likely to frighten clients. In his review of the existing literature, Fisher (2004) concluded this form of self-disclosure is uncommon and generally considered unethical. He then listed problems that can and do arise with self-disclosure:

- it could harm clients and/or the therapeutic relationship;
- a clinician could unconsciously be using this disclosure as a boundary crossing to evaluate a client's willingness to progress to sexual activity;

- there is no way for a therapist to know if their message is received by the client in the way in which it was intended, particularly for clients with preexisting vulnerabilities and difficulty with boundaries; and
- it could be used as supportive evidence in formal complaints against a professional.

At present, self-disclosure of sexual attraction to a client remains under-examined in the research, and much of it is based on personal opinion and case studies. Still, there is a consensus that this should be a rare occurrence and one that has been thoroughly processed through self-assessment, supervision, and consultation. In their work on the topic, Harris and Timm (2014) state,

> If you are the one attracted to your client, we still say, 'talk openly about it' … but do so in supervision. If you've developed an attraction to a client, you must remember that this is something *you* have to deal with.
>
> (p. 127)

The primary consideration must always be its impact on the involved client. Even those who suggest that it is indeed possible, such as above-mentioned Giovazolias and Davis (2001) as well as Marshall and Milton (2014), voice reservations. According to the latter,

> Where self-disclosure of a therapist's sexual feelings is chosen, it can be construed as a way of being genuine, ethical and authentic with the client's best interest at heart. However, therapists would be encouraged to critically think about the possibility that every good therapist's intention does not necessarily produce a positive outcome.
>
> (p. 222)

Conclusions

At this phase of the Boundary Violation Cycle Finally, a professional has typically recognized their romantic and sexual attraction to a client yet chooses to progress along the cycle. For the predatory type, the use of grooming and seduction via boundary crossings of ever-increasing intimacy is their modus operandi. For others of a non-predatory nature who are often overwhelmed by circumstances, including their own emotions, use of boundary crossings is a way to evaluate whether a client feels the same about them in a circumspect manner. Each reciprocated boundary crossing is a source of excitement leading to anticipation of further enticing intimacy. Finally, there are clinicians who completely repress, ignore, or minimize their attraction to a client; use of self-reflection and the assessments noted in this chapter might lead to the first glimmer of insight as to true motivating factors.

Consultation and supervision are needed at this point. Self-deception, distorted thinking, the AVE, and entrapment converge into one another leading to poor decision-making, often ignoring long-term repercussions in favor of short-term pleasure. Boundary crossings will escalate, including self-disclosure of attraction, and a person who has traversed along the cycle to this phase is at extremely high risk for a sexual boundary violation.

Summary

- Every mental health association recognizes sexual contact with a client is a boundary violation.
- Boundary crossings are departures from commonly accepted clinical practice that may or may not benefit the clients. Boundary crossing can be beneficial, neutral, or harmful to a client or the therapeutic process dependent on the circumstances.
- Boundary violations are departures from accepted practice that place the client or the therapeutic process at serious risk.
- Professional sexual violations are almost always preceded by a series of boundary crossings, including behaviors and interactions that in the beginning appear to have nothing to do with sex.
- The most common boundary crossing preceding sexual contact between clinician and patient is self-disclosure by the former.
- Several ethical principles guide decision-making as to whether a boundary crossing is in the best interests of a client:

  o Abstinence – Mental health professionals refrain from seeking personal gratification other than which is derived from being a part of the therapeutic process.
  o Neutrality – The client's agenda is the primary consideration in therapy.
  o Autonomy and independence – Professionals should not engage in activities that restrict these qualities.

- Researchers have formulated typologies of boundary crossings and violations, and many non-sexual boundary crossings preceding sexual violations have been delineated.
- In spite of known consequences, mental health professionals continue to engage in escalating boundary crossings for three reasons:
  - the AVE predicts that once a self-imposed promise regarding behavior has been broken, individuals can more easily continue on a path contrary to their promises;
  - entrapment occurs when they continues to invest in an unfavorable situation rather than ending it due to resources previously invested; and
  - cognitive distortions facilitate the process.
- Professionals engage in self-deception regarding boundary crossings and may not recognize they are occurring. This necessitates reliance on more objective forms of introspection and reflection, typically self-assessment, consultation, and supervision.
- The goal of self-assessment, consultation, and supervision is corrective action. A professional stops engaging in boundary crossings and judiciously changes course in the therapy process with the indicated client before an irrevocable boundary violation occurs.
- Self-disclosure of attraction to a client is a rare occurrence and generally considered unethical by practitioners.

References

Boysen, G. A. (2010). Integrating implicit bias into counselor education. *Counselor Education and Supervision*, 49(4), 210–227.

Bridges, N. A. (1998). Teaching psychiatric trainees to respond to sexual and loving feelings. *Journal of Psychotherapy Practice and Research*, 7(3), 217–226.

Brockner, J., Rubin, J. Z., Fine, J., Hamilton, T. P., Thomas, B., & Turetsky, B. (1982). Factors affecting entrapment in escalating conflicts: The importance of timing. *Journal of Research in Personality*, 16(2), 247–266.

Epstein, R. S., & Simon, R. I. (1990). The Exploitation Index: An early warning indicator of boundary violations in psychotherapy. *Menninger Bulletin*, 54, 450–465.

Epstein, R. S., Simon, R. I., & Kay, G. G. (1992). Assessing boundary violations in psychotherapy: Survey results with the Exploitation Index. *Bulletin of the Menninger Clinic*, 56(2), 150–166.

Fisher, C. D. (2004). Ethical issues in therapy: Therapist self-disclosure of sexual feelings. *Ethics & Behavior*, 14(2), 105–121.

Freud, S., Strachey, J., Freud, A., & Richards, A. (1953). *The Standard Edition of the complete psychological works of Sigmund Freud: Tr. from the German*. London, Unkted Kingdom: Hogarth Press.

Giovazolias, T., & Davis, P. (2001). How common is sexual attraction towards clients? The experiences of sexual attraction of counselling psychologists toward their clients and its impact on the therapeutic process. *Counselling Psychology Quarterly, 14*(4), 281–286.

Goodyear, R. K., & Shumate, J. L. (1996). Perceived effects of therapist self-disclosure of attraction to clients. *Professional Psychology: Research and Practice, 27*(6), 613–616.

Gottlieb, M. C. (1993). Avoiding exploitive dual relationships: A decision-making model. *Psychotherapy: Theory, Research, Practice, Training, 30*(1), 41–48.

Gutheil, T. G., & Gabbard, G. O. (1993). The concept of boundaries in clinical practice: Theoretical and risk-management dimensions. *American Journal of Psychiatry, 150*, 188–196.

Hamilton, J. C., & Spruill, J. (1999). Identifying and reducing risk factors related to trainee–Client sexual misconduct. *Professional Psychology: Research and Practice, 30*(3), 318–327.

Harris, S. M., & Timm, T. M. (2014). Sexual attraction in conjoint couple therapy. In M. Luca (Ed.), *Sexual attraction in therapy: Clinical perspectives on moving beyond the taboo* (pp. 115–130). West Sussex, UK: John Wiley & Sons.

Katz, J., Tirone, V., & Schukrafft, M. (2012). Breaking up is hard to do: Psychological entrapment and women's commitment to violent dating relationships. *Violence and Victims, 27*(4), 455–469.

Ladany, N., O'Brien, K. M., Hill, C. E., Melincoff, D. S., Knox, S., & Petersen, D. A. (1997). Sexual attraction toward clients, use of supervision, and prior training: A qualitative study of predoctoral psychology interns. *Journal of Counseling Psychology, 44*(4), 413–424.

Lamb, D. H., Catanzaro, S. J., & Moorman, A. S. (2003). Psychologists reflect on their sexual relationships with clients, supervisees, and students: Occurrence, impact, rationales and collegial intervention. *Professional Psychology: Research and Practice, 34*(1), 102.

Luca, M., & Boyden, M. (2014). An elephant in the room: A grounded theory of experienced psychotherapists' reactions and attitudes to sexual attraction. In M. Luca (Ed.), *Sexual attraction in therapy: Clinical perspectives on moving beyond the taboo* (pp. 193–208). West Sussex, UK: John Wiley & Sons.

Marlatt, G. A., & Gordon, J. R. (1985). *Relapse prevention: Maintenance strategies in the treatment of addictive behavior*. New York: Guilford Press.

Marshall, A., & Milton, M. (2014). Therapists' disclosures of their sexual feelings to their clients: The importance of honesty – An interpretative phenomenological approach. In M. Luca (Ed.), *Sexual attraction in therapy: Clinical perspectives on moving beyond the taboo* (pp. 209–225). West Sussex, UK: John Wiley & Sons.

Plaut, S. M. (2008). Sexual and nonsexual boundaries in professional relationships: Principles and teaching guidelines. *Sexual and Relationship Therapy, 23*(1), 85–94.

Pope, K. S. (1994). *Sexual involvement with therapists*. Washington, DC: American Psychological Association.

Pope, K. S., & Keith-Spiegel, P. (2008). A practical approach to boundaries in psychotherapy: Making decisions, bypassing blunders, and mending fences. *Journal of Clinical Psychology, 64*(5), 638–652.

Pope, K. S., Tabachnick, B. G., & Keith-Spiegel, P. (1987). Ethics of practice: The beliefs and behaviors of psychologists as therapists. *American Psychologist, 42*, 993–1006.

Sawyer, S., & Prescott, D. (2011). Boundaries and dual relationships. *Sexual Abuse, 23*(3), 365–380.

Simon, R. I. (1991). Psychological injury caused by boundary violation precursors to therapist-patient sex. *Psychiatric Annals, 21*(10), 614–619.

Simon, R. I. (1995). The natural history of therapist sexual misconduct: Identification and prevention. *Psychiatric Annals, 25*(2), 90–94.

Smith, D., & Fitzpatrick, M. (1995). Patient-therapist boundary issues: An integrative review of theory and research. *Professional Psychology: Research and Practice, 26*(5), 499–506.

Somer, E., & Saadon, M. (1999). Therapist-client sex: Clients' retrospective reports. *Professional Psychology: Research and Practice, 30*(5), 504–509.

Stake, J. E., & Oliver, J. (1991). Sexual contact and touching between therapist and client: A survey of psychologists' attitudes and behavior. *Professional Psychology: Research and Practice, 22*(4), 297–307.

Tschan, W. (2014). *Professional sexual misconduct in institutions: Causes and consequences, prevention and intervention.* Boston, MA: Hogrefe Publishing.

Wheeler, J. G., George, W. H., & Marlatt, G. A. (2006). Relapse prevention for sexual offenders: Considerations for the "abstinence violation effect". *Sexual Abuse, 18*(3), 233–248.

Violations and Post-Violation Considerations

8

At this point on the Boundary Violation Cycle a clinician has progressed from the triggering of a romantically or sexually appealing client onto fantasies, permissive self-talk, and non-sexual boundary crossings. They have allowed internal boundaries, such as knowledge of consequences, to erode while simultaneously manipulating the environment and client so as to advance a goal of fulfillment of sexual desire. Step by step, therapeutic neutrality disintegrates. Many offending professionals also fall in love with a client. Regardless, at some point an actual sexual event occurs.

Celenza (2007) defines a professional boundary violation as any kind of physical contact occurring within the confines of therapeutic relationship for the purpose of erotic pleasure. However, this definition is delimiting because it elides non-contact behaviors that are nonetheless violations. Halter, Brown, and Stone (2007), in their exhaustive review of research on sexual boundary violations by health professionals described the behavior thusly:

> Clinical and therapeutic interventions inevitably render individual patients and clients vulnerable, and trust relies on providing a safe and boundaried space in which these can be carried out without compromising the person's dignity and bodily integrity. Sexual boundary violations occur wherever a clinical or therapeutic relationship is turned into a sexual or sexualised encounter.
>
> (p. 11)

Tschan (2013) offered a more comprehensive definition, which he states is as any form of sexualized behavior committed within a professional role whether a client consents or even initiates the process. He then offered three categories of sexual behavior.

- (Attempted) penetration (vaginal, anal, oral), genital stimulation; whether with or without ejaculation or orgasm (hands-on).
- Sexual impropriety – such as kissing, fondling, taking pictures of intimate body parts – including voyeuristic or exhibitionistic behavior, and presenting pornographic material (hands-off).
- Dating or attempted dating.

Tschan also reminds us that high profile cases too often mislead the field into thinking that a boundary violation equates to "penis in vagina," which has three unintended consequences. First, it allows us to elide other serious offenses – such as a professional masturbating in front of a client or sending homemade pornography to the latter – as though these are somehow less serious and possibly even deserving of less severe consequences when discovered. Second, it allows offending clinicians to minimize the seriousness of their actions by rationalizing "Nothing really serious happened" because penetration did not occur. Finally, it negates the experience of female professionals who engage in boundary violations, and likewise ignores same-sex sexual behaviors.

Let's re-visit Jessica and her client Joseph. Boundary crossings have at this point become frequent. Texts and telephone calls about non-clinical topics occur frequently, and the romantic and sexual chemistry between the two of them is obvious to both. Neither has outright stated it though. Jessica, ashamed of her behavior, does not seek out supervision or colleague input. Instead, she argues with herself; a recognition and acknowledgment of the inappropriateness of her behavior struggles with her desire for Joseph. Still, she is able to rationalize and justify every action that further blurs their boundaries. Her most common refrain is, "What am I doing?"

Jessica passively continues on this pathway until they decide to meet for a drink on a weekend night. Three drinks into this meeting they are holding hands and professing their attraction to one another. As Joseph drives her back to her apartment, their hands meet, and before she exits the car, they engage in a highly charged kiss lasting several minutes. He also strokes her breasts. As she enters her apartment panic sets in. "What am I going to do? Do I need to stop seeing him as a patient? How can I explain this need to end his treatment to my supervisor? Will Joseph tell his friends about me, which may somehow get back to my employer? My God! I just destroyed my career," she tells herself. She then begins to strategize as to how to keep this a secret until she can figure out what she should do.

The remainder of this chapter examines what happens after a boundary violation occurs. A professional recognizes they have engaged in a serious breach of conduct that could be catastrophic for all involved. How does the person handle this situation?

Post-Violation Considerations

Models espousing a cyclical approach to problematic behavior agree there is a post-behavior phase. For example, all such models of sex offending describe a "post-offending phase," such as in the work of Kahn (1990), who formulated a four-phase cycle, the last of which is called the pretend normal phase, in which offenders return to a normal routine and act as if the offense never occurred. Ward, Louden, Hudson, and Marshall (1995) found that many post-offending individuals feel guilt, remorse, and regret, and even resolve to never repeat the act.

Following a boundary violation, a professional too is left to determine how to respond. Three concerns typically occur simultaneously. First, he must grapple with his own reactions to the violation, which are often a conflux of guilt, fear, excitement, relief, and, in many cases, anticipation of further sexual/romantic involvement with the indicated client. Second, the professional must also manage the reactions of the client, who is likely experiencing a similar combination of thoughts and emotions as the professional. Finally, there is a continued need to keep others from learning about the violation, which requires further manipulation of the environment as well as friends, colleagues, and family.

In general there are two options for professionals engaging in a sexual boundary violation: either end the behavior or continue it. Both paths necessitate continued secrecy. Gartrell, Herman, Olarte, Feldstein, and Localio (1988) remind us, "Because of the private and undocumented nature of sexual contact between a therapist and a patient ... it comes to attention of others only if disclosed by the patient or the offending therapist" (p. 1070).

Continuation of the Sexual/Romantic Relationship

Obviously the best choice for a transgressing professional would be to stop the behavior, but the numerous psychological principles already noted in this text – distorted self-talk, the impact of arousal on problem solving, entrapment, the AVE, and at this point, fear of consequences – inform us that this is unlikely. Having fallen in love with a client adds even more complications.

Professionals who continue the behavior attempt to depict normalcy in their lives and present as unchanged in any way to friends, family, and colleagues. Through the use of distorted thinking they minimize the possibility of discovery and convince themselves that they can get away with the relationship. In other cases, the clinician recognizes that attempting to end or curtail a relationship with a client could lead the latter to disclose the activity; fear of consequences leads them to continue even if they would sincerely like to stop. Both professional and client actively engage in obfuscating their relationship so as to protect themselves.

Another consideration is whether the professional relationship must end. Some professionals attempt a romantic/sexual relationship with a client while continuing to treat them, while others believe that ending treatment justifies continued romantic/sexual involvement. A common misconception in the mental health field is that it is permissible to maintain a romantic/sexual relationship with a patient if the therapeutic one comes to an end. Berkman, Turner, Cooper, Polnerow, and Swartz (2000) assessed master's level social workers' attitudes and educational preparation regarding sexual contact with clients and found that between 30% and 35% of respondents approved of sexual contact in situations where professional relationships were terminated more than 5 years ago, were less than two sessions, or had involved only limited or concrete services. Mattison, Jayaratne, and Croxton (2002) identified a current lack of consensus in the social work profession regarding the definition of an "ex-client." In a survey of 654 randomly selected social workers practicing in the US, 46.8% stated that a client is always a client while 40.9% said the client becomes an ex-client at the point of termination. The remaining 12.1% gave their own specific time period ranging from 6 months to 10 years. Shavit and Bucky (2004) interviewed psychologists and found consensus that termination of treatment did not resolve transference and countertransference issues and therefore opposed the concept of terminating the therapeutic relationship in order to enter into a sexual relationship.

One final outcome is that a professional ultimately – typically after an extended period of pretend normal – relinquishes their career in order to maintain a sexual or romantic relationship with a client. This appears to be a most uncommon outcome.

There is scant research on the relationship dynamics between professionals and patients who continue a romantic relationship, whether this includes continued therapeutic involvement or not. Common sense would dictate that the secretiveness, duplicity, shifting power differentials, and underlying mental health issues for the client and professional would lead them to be short-lived. Somer and Saadon (1999) interviewed patients who had been involved in sexual relationships with therapists. They found the duration of the sexual affairs ranged from a single incident of sexual contact to a 96-month relationship that was still ongoing when the data were collected; the average duration of the sexual liaisons was 10.2 months. 48% of the respondents expressed current anger at their former therapists, 37% still felt guilt and shame over the affairs, and 19% expressed current feelings of disappointment and disillusionment about their unfortunate therapeutic experiences. Lamb, Catanzaro, and Moorman (2003) asked psychologists who had engaged in prohibited sexual relationships with clients, supervisees, and students to reflect on the impact associated with engaging in such relationships. The sexual relationships established typically did not last for a very long time, and the course of the relationship was not always positive. One half of the involved psychologists reported the relationship was not worth having. McNulty, Ogden, and Warren (2013) similarly interviewed mental health professionals who had publicly been found in breach of professional standards because of sexual contact with a client or ex-client. They found that these relationships failed, often because of a re-emergence of the client's mental health problems. These clients, whose initial symptoms had seemed mild, amenable to treatment, and which seemed ostensibly resolved before initiation of a romantic or sexual relationship, were later portrayed during the relationship as "dramatic images of madness and instability; [needing] inpatient admissions, [and] Jeckyll and Hyde unpredictability" (p 193). Clinicians also expressed resentment towards these clients and identified them as manipulative. Nachmani and Somer (2007) interviewed women who had been sexually involved with their therapist and reported sexual contact spanned an average of 41 sessions, and, truly a disturbing feature, more than half continued to pay for sessions even after sexual contact occurred. 61% of the participants reported they terminated the sexual relationship.

Ending of the Sexual/Romantic Relationship

Clinicians can also stop the violating behavior, and here one of two common scenarios usually occurs. First, a clinician stops the behavior but tries to continue to work with the client in a therapeutic fashion. As stated above, research on such dynamics is almost non-existent due to the secretiveness of the behavior. The majority of those in the mental health field would attest that damage to the therapeutic process wrought by a boundary violation is irreversible.

However, attempts to maintain the process occur for a number of reasons. Likely paramount of them all, is a clinician's fear of consequences. To end a sexual and treatment relationship might lead a client to reveal a violation. Another likely scenario is that the client does not want to end the therapeutic involvement. Recall that many clients enter treatment naïve as to the process and what it entails. They have likely bonded with a counselor and the loss of this seemingly trustworthy person is yet another trauma in their lives. Somer and Nachmani (2005) interviewed individuals who had had sexual contact with their therapist; all reported a high level of dependency on the offending therapists and that the ending of the relationship led to guilt, confusion, and deterioration of their mental health. Disch and Avery (2001) examined the emotional experiences of individuals who had experienced therapist–client sex. The majority reported feeling special and taken care of; approximately half reported feeling loved and being in love while the relationship was occurring. Disch (2006) interviewed women who had been abused by a professional and determined they entered treatment with significant histories of victimization. Nachmani and Somer (2007) found clients idealized professionals before and often during a sexual relationship; words such as "God, guru, prophet, savior, angel" were some of the descriptors used (p. 7). Many of the women reported feeling privileged that a therapist had chosen them for a partner. These studies in sum indicate that ending of a therapeutic relationship may present as overwhelming and one that patients may resist. This becomes even more complex for individuals who were already involved in a romantic relationship with another partner prior to the boundary violation.

Second, professionals may end the romantic relationship and therapy relationship altogether. They may attempt to pacify a client's concerns and minimize risk of disclosure. However, if mental health concerns are still evident, they may initiate a transfer to another clinician asking them to promise not to reveal the underlying circumstances leading to this change. Still, disclosure to a new treatment provider remains one of the primary methods by which we learn about boundary violations. Those engaged in this behavior recognize this and are reluctant to refer to a new provider.

Summary of Post-Violation Considerations

Relationships between professionals and patients seem to be short-lived, end poorly, and have emotional ramifications for both parties. Patients are often the person to end them. There is also a need for secrecy, whether one makes efforts to end or continue a relationship. Even for those rare professionals who voluntarily leave the field to remain in a romantic/sexual relationship, efforts are made to hide the true genesis of the couple.

There is only one option that allows professionals to avoid the need for secrecy: voluntarily disclosure. Professionals engaging in boundary violations can self-report to colleagues, supervisors, the agencies in which they work, and to licensing and certification boards. These individuals acknowledge the inappropriateness of their actions, the harm occurring to the involved patient(s), and are accepting of consequences. While this does occur, there are no accurate statistics indicating the frequency. It is likely a rare occurrence though due to consequences, most often severe punitive actions such as revocation of a license, expulsion from professional membership, and formal public censure. Illustrating the upheaval that comes with self-disclosure, Celenza (2007) concludes the process is traumatic, the professional suffers immensely, and that many can be driven to the point of suicide.

Conclusions

Boundary violations occur by dating clients or engaging in sexual behavior with them, including non-contact sexual interactions. Once a sexual boundary violation occurs, the relationship with the involved client is permanently altered. During the Post-Violation Considerations Stage clinicians must decide how to respond knowing all the while that secrecy is paramount and that their careers are in jeopardy. Repercussions include revocation of a license, expulsion from professional membership, and formal public censure.

Professionals must now consider how to interact with the involved client in light of the changed dynamics of their relationship. A minority of clinicians may voluntarily disclose their behavior to authorities. In most cases though, clinicians attempt to either continue the relationship, even attempting to continue therapy with the client, or end the relationship (and possibly even therapy) and engage in damage control. Regardless, the relationship between the professional and counselor now harbors secretiveness, duplicity, and shifting power differentials; mental health problems also tend to rebound. Romantic/sexual relationships between counselors and clients tend to be short lived and end poorly; often the latter initiates the end of the relationship. Clinical neutrality is also no longer a realistic option and harm to the client is the typical outcome.

Summary

- Sexual boundary violations occur when a clinical or therapeutic relationship is turned into a sexual or sexualized encounter. It includes physical and non-physical contact as well as dating.
- During the post-sexual violation stage, a professional copes with their own reactions, the reactions of the involved client, and makes active attempts to hide the activity from friends, colleagues, and family.
- There are two options for professionals engaging in a sexual boundary violation: either end the behavior or continue it.
- For those choosing to continue the relationship, some professionals also attempt to continue therapy. Some stop meeting with the client as a therapist. Others relinquish their career in order to maintain a sexual or romantic relationship with a client.
- Relationships between professionals and patients seem to be short-lived, end poorly, and have emotional ramifications for both parties.
- For those choosing to end the relationship, some professionals attempt to realign therapeutic boundaries even though damage to the therapeutic process wrought by a sexual violation is irreversible.
- Professionals may end the romantic relationship and therapy relationship altogether.

References

Berkman, C. S., Turner, S. G., Cooper, M., Polnerow, D., & Swartz, M. (2000). Sexual contact with clients: Assessment of social workers' attitudes and educational preparation. *Social Work, 45*(3), 223–235.

Celenza, A. (2007). *Sexual boundary violations*. Lanham, MD: Jason Aronson.

Disch, E. (2006). Sexual victimization and revictimization of women by professionals: Client experiences and implications for subsequent treatment. *Women & Therapy, 29*(1–2), 41–61.

Disch, E., & Avery, N. (2001). Sex in the consulting room, the examining room, and the sacristy: Survivors of sexual abuse by professionals. *American Journal of Orthopsychiatry, 71*(2), 204–217.

Gartrell, N., Herman, J. L., Olarte, S., Feldstein, M., & Localio, R. (1988). Management and rehabilitation of sexually exploitive therapists. *Psychiatric Services, 39*(10), 1070–1074.

Halter, M., Brown, H., & Stone, J. (2007). Sexual boundary violations by health professionals–An overview of the published empirical literature. Council for Healthcare Regulatory Excellence.

Kahn, T. J. (1990). *Pathways: A guided workbook for youth beginning treatment.* Orwell, VT: Safer Society Press.

Lamb, D. H., Catanzaro, S. J., & Moorman, A. S. (2003). Psychologists reflect on their sexual relationships with clients, supervisees, and students: Occurrence, impact, rationales and collegial intervention. *Professional Psychology: Research and Practice, 34*(1), 102–107.

Mattison, D., Jayaratne, S., & Croxton, T. (2002). Client or former client? Implications of ex-client definition on social work practice. *Social Work, 47*(1), 55–64.

McNulty, N., Ogden, J., & Warren, F. (2013). 'Neutralizing the patient': Therapists' accounts of sexual boundary violations. *Clinical Psychology & Psychotherapy, 20*(3), 189–198.

Nachmani, I., & Somer, E. (2007). Women sexually victimized in psychotherapy speak out: The dynamics and outcome of therapist-client sex. *Women & Therapy, 30*(1–2), 1–17.

Shavit, N., & Bucky, S. (2004). Sexual contact between psychologists and their former therapy patients: Psychoanalytic perspectives and professional implications. *American Journal of Psychoanalysis, 64*(3), 229–248.

Somer, E., & Nachmanil, I. (2005). Constructions of therapist-client sex: A comparative analysis of retrospective victim reports. *Sexual Abuse: Journal of Research & Treatment, 17*(1), 47–62.

Somer, E., & Saadon, M. (1999). Therapist-client sex: Clients' retrospective reports. *Professional Psychology: Research and Practice, 30*(5), 504–509.

Tschan, W. (2013). *Professional sexual misconduct in institutions: Causes and consequences, prevention and intervention.* Boston: Hogrefe Publishing.

Ward, T., Louden, K., Hudson, S. M., & Marshall, W. L. (1995). A descriptive model of the offense chain for child molesters. *Journal of Interpersonal Violence, 10*(4), 452–472.

Education, Training, and Supervision

9

Education, training, and supervision are well recognized as preventative measures for sexual boundary violations. What is also recognized is that their true potential is underutilized. Mental health workers receive very few hours of formal training on the topic of sexual attraction in therapy, and that which is obtained is of indeterminate quality. We already know sexual boundary violations are harmful and destructive, a point that is reiterated throughout our careers; yet this is the extent of the education most of us receive on the topic. Even supervision, the one venue which is most recommended for addressing sexual feelings in clinical work, does not adequately (if at all) address the topic. There is a myriad of reasons for these glaring deficits as well as numerous cogent recommendations for improving upon them. These will be explored in this chapter.

As a starting point though it must be made clear that education and supervision are mutually reinforcing. We cannot have quality supervision on sexual feelings in treatment until supervisors have quality education on the topic.

College and University Education

Preparing students for management of sexual attraction to clients is a cornerstone in prevention efforts. In the 1990s, as research on professional boundary violations began to proliferate, there were clear edicts to begin instructing therapists early in their careers about appropriate treatment boundaries (e.g., Simon, 1995). Two decades later, in one of the most exhaustive reviews of professional boundary violation research, Halter, Brown, and Stone (2007) determined those who receive education on the topic are less likely to violate.

In spite of the consensus that formal education regarding boundary violations is a necessary component in prevention, several challenges have been noted. First, the majority of practicing professionals report that their formal university training did not prepare them for sexual arousal in the clinical realm. Bernsen, Tabachnick, and Pope (1994), in a poll of social workers, found that the majority reported receiving no graduate training on sexual attraction. Paxton, Lovett, and Riggs (2001) surveyed 293 university-based therapists and found a similar pattern: the majority of the respondents did not have specific learning opportunities in their graduate-level training programs related to ethical and therapeutic management of sexual feelings in working with clients. Pope, Keith-Spiegel, and Tabachnick (2006) surveyed psychotherapists about experiences of sexual attraction to clients. Responses indicated that half of the respondents did not receive any guidance or training concerning this issue, and only 9% reported that their training or supervision was adequate.

A second challenge concerns the quality of education students receive regarding sexual boundaries. Housman and Stake (1999) mailed questionnaires to the directors of clinical psychology doctoral programs and six students in each program to measure the amount of training in sexual ethics provided. In addition, students were asked to respond to a sexual ethics vignette. While the researchers found that nearly all programs participating in the survey (many of those queried did not respond to the invitation to participate) provided sexual ethics training, many students still did not grasp their significance. For example, 7% of the students in the present study did not know that sex with current clients is always prohibited, 34% did not understand that termination or transfer does not free therapists to have sex with their clients, and 68% did not know that sexual feelings for clients are normal and not unethical. The researchers determined that while increasing the number of course hours allotted to sexual ethics is important, so too is making the material more effective.

Unfortunately, there is no clear consensus as to what boundary training in formal education should consist of. While there are numerous suggestions as to the content and number of hours comprising such trainings, very few have undergone any form of rigorous evaluation. Vasquez (1988) suggests that ethics trainings for students should emphasize the violations most likely to occur in the field, which includes sexual contact in clinical settings. She states, "Students have a right to know the consequences of unethical behavior ahead of time" (p. 68). Students, she proposes, should increase understanding of the psychology of men and women, gender socialization, sexualization of relationships, legal and professional consequences, and harm to clients. Self-awareness arising from feedback, dialogue, and role-plays and other experiential activities help students recognize blind spots and personal risk factors. Finally, training programs must occur in environments that promote ethical behavior; most important is that faculty model ethical behavior and support explorations of sexual topics likely to occur during the course of professionals' careers. The author also reminds us that training programs have an obligation to prevent those who are unsuitable from entering the field. Similarly, Strasburger, Jorgenson, and Sutherland (1992) advise that universities do a better job at screening applicants and those found unfit for mental health practice should be removed as early as possible. They also suggest trainees be taught to anticipate when the intensity of the therapeutic relationship requires seeking supervision or consultation.

Seto (1995) suggests ethical decision-making should be emphasized throughout one's entire university training instead of being limited to a single semester on ethics and professional issues, as is typical in graduate programs. In addition to the topics mentioned above, he also promotes exploration of transference and countertransference, normalizing the experience of sexual attraction in therapy, and self-management strategies. Housman and Stake (1999) urge that training programs consider augmented training for male students based on their increased risk for engagement in professional sexual boundary violations, particularly examining gender roles and expectations implicitly and explicitly held by these budding professionals. Pope et al. (2006) suggest that textbooks should reflect sexual attraction in therapy issues though they admit such resources are rare or that the topic is mentioned in only a cursory manner. Fronek et al. (2009) stressed the unique issues for rural populations be considered, including the likelihood that boundary crossings would occur (e.g., a patient is also the only plumber in the community so there may be a higher chance of meeting outside the clinical setting). Finally, Steinberg and Alpert (2017) suggest attention be paid to post-termination relationships as this is a time when many clinicians feel it is safer and less ethically egregious to engage in boundary crossings.

We must also consider the clinical placements of students, which is a requirement for graduate programs. Students may inadvertently be placed in facilities as part of their internship where unethical practices reign and/or have interactions with colleagues and supervisors in which suggestions, advice, and directives contrary to those taught in their education-based programs are proffered. Students may directly encounter dual relationships, sexualized relationships, and even professional boundary crossings between staff and patients as well as supervisors and their employees. They may unfortunately be working in a facility in which sexual violation becomes known and witness unhealthy organizational responses (e.g., actively conspiring to minimize the chance the incident is reported to authorities) and victim blaming, in which colleagues hold the involved client as culpable for the sexual activity that occurred with the participating clinician.

There is also growing acknowledgment that sexual attraction should be part of a much more extensive and thorough curriculum for graduate students on sex and sexuality, and, according to Hamilton and Spruill (1999), the earlier in one's career this happens, the better the outcome; in all cases, they argue, the topic must be addressed before students begin working with clients. They then offered a list of topics that should be covered, including:

- the powerful effects of attraction;
- personal accounts by professionals regarding their experience with attraction in clinical settings;
- risk factors and early warning signs of an impending boundary violation, such as escalating boundary crossings;
- steps to follow when attraction occurs, particularly seeking supervision;
- consequences of a sexual boundary violation, particularly its impact on a client; and
- a discussion of the university's policy on boundary crossings and violations.

Ford and Hendrick (2003) developed a curriculum ideally suited to a weekly 1–2 hour seminar occurring during a student's practicum or internship. However, in contrast to above-mentioned Hamilton and Spruill (1999), they propose it should be part of a comprehensive package of sexual issues and problems common in the field. Becoming comfortable with sexual topics is an essential skill for clinicians since they will frequently manifest in one form or another as part of clients' presenting problems. Thus in addition to addressing sexual attraction in therapy and effective use of sexual transference, a thorough curriculum also reviews common presenting sexual problems, sexual preferences and practices, sexual dysfunctions, sexuality across the lifespan, sex therapy methods and techniques, and nontraditional sexual practices.

Few outcome studies of university-based trainings exist, a point noted in Halter, Brown, and Stone's (2007) review of the research, which located only two such studies for those in mental health practice.

Summary of College and University-Based Interventions

While more education programs are including sexual topics in their ethics and professional development courses, it is unclear how far we have advanced since 1999, when Housman and Stake reviewed existing research and determined that between 33% and 55% of professionals reported receiving no training in sexual ethics in their graduate programs. It is doubtless that many graduate students continue to receive inadequate preparation as part of their graduate education. A lack of consensus regarding the range of topics that should be subsumed, sequencing of delivery, training modalities (e.g., didactic presentations vs. role plays), assessment, and outcome evaluation remain problematic. Well-developed, meaningful, and effective efforts are more of an aspiration than a reality.

In sum though, there is without doubt an agreement that trainings programs should model ethical behavior, be staffed by individuals comfortable with sexual topics, use a variety of approaches to address an often-contentious topic, focus on increasing self-awareness of risk potential for sexual boundary violations, and normalize sexual feelings in treatment. Paxton et al. (2001), in their interviews with psychotherapists, found that those who had access to the following learning opportunities rated their graduate-level training related to sexual feelings in therapy as better in comparison to those who did not have these opportunities:

- The availability of supervisors who were perceived by the respondents to agree that sexual feelings are a natural, expected part of any human relationship.
- Content-specific ethics courses which included an opportunity to explore ways in which the respondent might react to feelings of sexual attraction to a client. This topic was not however constrained to one course, and sexual topics were or could be addressed in other classes.
- An opportunity to explore one's sexual values, attitudes, and beliefs.

The above authors also found that postgraduate training on responding to sexual feelings in therapy and exploring attitudes and beliefs made a significant difference in participants' careers, a topic to which we now turn.

Continuing Education

Nearly every jurisdiction that issues a license or certification to practice in the mental health field requires continuing education courses for renewal. These continuing education requirements vary from one jurisdiction to another, from the number of hours required to the types of courses that must be taken. All however require a minimal number of hours specifically related to ethics. Common topics in these trainings regardless of one's professional title include confidentiality, mandated reporting, informed consent, and dual relationships. Sexual boundary violations are often subsumed under the latter topic. Continuing education courses typically occur via grand rounds presentations, articles in journals, workshops, and home-study courses.

Professionals participating in continuing education are already aware that sexual and romantic behavior between themselves and clients is contraindicated, and trainings typically merely remind participants that the behavior is harmful to all involved, can destroy one's career and reputation, and advise addressing the topic with a supervisor. Pope et al. (2006) note however that reliance on sanctions and fear of consequences has not proven particularly effective in stemming sexual boundary violations. Another challenge is those who have been practicing in the field for an extended period of time may believe they are resistant or even immune to sexual attraction and the risk of dual relationships though it is clear that length of time in the field by no means protects against the behavior. As a result of the above challenges, many professionals are dismissive of, or outright avoid, such trainings. After all, they already know sexual boundary violations are unethical, have consequences, and have either successfully dealt with attraction in clinical settings in the past or not yet experienced it; why then, they ask themselves, do I need a training on the topic? Training takes time away from an already hectic schedule, and the majority of professionals want to attend a topic that they would find valuable. Too many believe they already know enough about the topic of sexual boundary violations.

The quality of continuing education presents with another challenge. It is possible at the present time to take an ethics continuing education course that condenses the topic of sexual and romantic relationship with clients into mere minutes or, in a home-study format, several paragraphs, which nonetheless meets a jurisdiction's requirements for ethics training. These are by no means comprehensive trainings. However, the content of a "comprehensive" training on the topic has not been formalized, and even those offering a several hour or multi-day training on the specific topic approach it differently dependent on the provider. At present, two themes buttress most available trainings. First, sexual and romantic attraction in clinical settings is normal and to be expected. Second, there are healthy and unhealthy methods of dealing with these feelings. The following several paragraphs describe recommendations in the research for topics to be covered in trainings on sexual boundary violations.

Fronek et al. (2009) determined that any training on boundary violations should include a component on general ethical-decision making and recommended use of a five-step ethical decision making model.

1. Define the problem.
2. What guidelines/rules already exist?

3. Identify and consider the options (inclusive of critical reflection, consultation or supervision).
4. Test the options (inclusive of critical reflection, consultation or supervision).
5. Choose your course of action (inclusive of critical reflection, consultation or supervision).

Similarly, Pope and Keith-Spiegel (2008) outline that any training on the topic of sexual boundary violations should begin with the introduction of a decision-making matrix for boundary crossings, which includes the following considerations:

*   Imagine what might be the "best possible outcome" and the "worst possible outcome" from both crossing this boundary and from not crossing this boundary.
*   Consider the research and other published literature on this boundary crossing.
*   Be familiar with and take into account any guidance regarding this boundary crossing offered by professional guidelines, ethics codes, legislation, case law, and other resources.
*   Identify at least one colleague you can trust for honest feedback on boundary crossing questions.
*   Pay attention to any uneasy feelings, doubts, or confusions – try to figure out what's causing them and what implications, if any, they may have for your decisions.
*   At the start of therapy and as part of informed consent, describe to the client exactly how you work and what kind of psychotherapy you do.
*   Keep careful notes on any planned boundary crossing, describing exactly why, in your clinical judgment, this was (or will be) helpful to the client.

Tschan (2014) recommends post-graduate trainings encompass personal risk assessment, including proximal, distal, environmental, and client factors. Building on this, some trainings teach individuals self-monitoring techniques, including use of self-assessments, such as the Epstein and Simon (1990) Exploitation Index, a self-assessment questionnaire developed for therapists to identify early warning indicators of boundary violations introduced in Chapter 7. Celenza (2007), a leader in the field, suggests trainings incorporate discussions of transference, power differentials, ethics, and clinician self-care. The Council for Healthcare Regulatory Excellence (2008) in the United Kingdom recommends use of lectures, case studies/vignettes, video enactments of problematic scenarios, small group activities, and workbooks examining topics such as:

- description of boundaries and their importance in clinical work;
- consequences of boundary violations for all involved, including collateral victims;
- examples of sexual boundary crossings, including interactions with former patients;
- unequal power dynamics in clinical relationships;
- the impact of sexual arousal on clinical judgment;
- acknowledging the signs of sexual attraction;
- management of a professional's attraction;
- management of a patient's attraction; and
- use of supervision and consultation.

Gabbard (1996), one of the vanguard leaders of boundary violations research, stated, "[I]f we don't police our own profession, others will do it for us" (p. 320). He determined that retrospective analysis of an incident almost always leads co-workers to acknowledge that something was amiss with a colleague who violated. However they rationalized that it was not their right to intrude on the privacy of the therapist–patient relationship. He thus urged professionals to empathically monitor each other. Twenty years later, Capawana (2016) concluded that comprehensive trainings must also teach participants to actively monitor colleagues' engagement with self-care practices, questionable therapeutic/supervisory dynamics, and power dynamics.

Summary of Continuing Education Interventions

As with college and university training, there is a consensus that postgraduate training on sexual boundary violations is an essential preventative method. Also similar to university-based settings is a lack of agreement as to what comprehensive training should consist of or how often it should occur. Starting with an acknowledgment that treatment providers already know boundary violations are wrong and have consequences, how do we then build upon this to create meaningful content? The research in this chapter offered several pertinent recommendations:

- include information on ethical-decision making;
- reiterate that sexual and romantic attraction is normal and to be expected and that there are healthy and unhealthy way to manage these feelings;

- educate participants as to the myriad of risk factors for a sexual boundary violation, that risk is dynamic and ever changing, and offer opportunities to engage in self-assessment;
- use self-care to reduce risk;
- introduce a model explaining that a sexual boundary violation is the end result of a process and does not just suddenly occur;
- implement management of a clinician's attraction;
- implement management of a client's attraction to the professional;
- use supervision and consultation; and
- engage in empathic monitoring of colleagues.

It is also unclear at this point which modalities are best suited for dissemination of the above topics, though most of the articles cited above support use of several concurrent methods, including small-group discussion, role plays, consideration of case vignettes, and didactic presentation. Fronek et al. (2009), as one example, reported positive participant feedback from a 1-day training on professional boundaries using a purposeful multidisciplinary approach consisting of doctors, nurses, physiotherapists, occupational therapists, social workers, psychologists, dietitians, and speech therapists. The cross-pollination of opinions and experiences were found to be particularly valuable by participants.

In sum, though we are unsure of the optimal training curriculum and delivery methods, we know enough now that all those in the field should be receiving more comprehensive training than is the current norm.

Enhanced Supervision

Murray and Sommers-Flanagan (2014) remind us that supervision is a "safety net for quality client care and the foundation for clinical skill development" (p. 104). Based on this appraisal, it is then the ideal setting to discuss sexual attraction to a client. Indeed, Paxton et al. (2001), in their surveys of practicing psychotherapists, determined those who had past supervisors willing to discuss sexual attraction in therapy reported they were better prepared for these occurrences. Still, innumerable studies conclude supervision for this topic does not consistently occur. Through recalling of past supervisory relationships, interviewing participants after a single supervisory session, or tracking supervisory experiences over time, it is apparent that supervisors and supervisees express reservations about addressing this topic. Supervisees offer many reasons for eliding this topic, including:

- the topic is perceived as unimportant;
- embarrassment;
- concern about its impact on the professional's image and status;
- a supervisor appears unapproachable or untrustworthy;
- a supervisor appears uncomfortable with sexual topics;
- a supervisor does not introduce the topic;
- fear of negative reaction by supervisor;
- fear of a negative evaluation;
- fear the one will be asked to transfer the client to another clinician; and
- impression management.

Ladany (2004) enumerated numerous obstacles to quality supervision. First, many supervisors receive little to no training for the position. Second, supervisors often use their own past experiences of supervision as guides for current behavior, which is particularly problematic if this supervision was lacking in quality. Also, supervisors are often far more comfortable using techniques and approaches recognized as essential for work with clients, such as a nonjudgmental stance, in contrast to critical feedback, which is essential for supervision. Finally, there are few available resources for evaluating psychotherapy skills. In regards to sexual attraction in clinical settings, many supervisors feel uncomfortable or unknowledgeable about the topic and, if it is addressed at all, simply remind practitioners of the consequences of acting on attraction. Supervisors are also unsure of the goals of discussing sexual attraction in therapy other than preventing a boundary violation; as pointed out in this book though working through attraction leads to insight, skills development, and conceptualization of its impact on the therapeutic process. Finally, supervisors are fearful that bringing up this topic could be misinterpreted by a supervisee as a sexual overture. If it becomes apparent that a supervisor is uncomfortable with a particular topic, a trainee or supervisee in turn may adjust their style to become more withholding, distort their experiences, or outright conceal their concerns; in short, they become less open and instead more guarded and hypervigilant (Gray, Ladany, Walker, & Ancis, 2001).

One last consideration is the dynamics of supervision. In most cases, supervision is involuntary; those working in treatment organizations are required to meet with a supervisor, whether they want to or not. Supervisees also rarely have input into their choice of a supervisor. These same supervisors evaluate their supervisee(s), a process that can impact graduation from a university program or promotions and raises in the workplace; power dynamics no doubt shape the outcome of supervision. Thus, with all of the above obstacles, is not surprising that Ladany (2007) concludes that effective supervision occurs less than half of the time and excellent supervision on a mere 11% of occasions.

Several recommendations have been formulated for increasing the likelihood that supervision will effectively address the topic of sexual attraction. First, supervisors must have a clear understanding of the rationale for introducing the topic into relationships with supervisees. Certainly prevention of harm to the client and collateral victims remains the paramount goal, but other considerations are also relevant. These include reassurances that feelings of attraction for a client are common and not a source of shame. Supervision can explore the impact of attraction on the treatment process. Recall that professionals can and do use attraction to facilitate treatment rather than instinctively disengaging from a client when it arises. Attraction can portend much meaning for a clinician too if explored in depth. Supervisees, for example, can come to understand their vulnerabilities and life dissatisfactions that place them at risk for a boundary violation. Finally, working through sexual attraction in supervision helps supervisees to learn and improve self-regulation skills (Luca & Boyden, 2014). Murray and Sommers-Flanagan (2014) suggest that supervisors openly address the importance of sexual attraction in clinical practice early in a relationship with a supervisee to indicate that the topic is not off-limits and then be broached throughout their work together as a reminder of its significance.

A second recommendation is that supervisors create an environment in which supervisee self-disclosure feels safe. Sexual attraction is just one of many topics that a supervisee might passively or actively avoid discussing during supervision, including clinical mistakes, personal issues interfering with treatment, and countertransference issues. There is a consensus that disclosure of these topics requires a strong supervisory working alliance that reduces anxiety and promotes self-efficacy (e.g., Ladany, 2014; Mehr, Ladany, & Caskie, 2015). Supervisors should use basic counseling skills such as listening, empathy, reflecting of feelings, and engaging in judicious and appropriate self-disclosure (Ladany, Mori, & Mehr, 2013). Supervisors should also be open to feedback, discuss power differentials, and specifically describe the evaluation process (Mehr, Ladany, & Caskie, 2010).

Finally, supervisors themselves must become comfortable with and knowledgeable about the presence of sexual attraction in therapy. Supervisees will elide the topic if they sense a supervisor is uncomfortable with it, incompetent to address it, or likely to shame them. Supervisory modeling of this delicate topic can be an example for supervisees when it arises with a client.

Summary of Enhanced Supervision

While the importance of supervision for preventing sexual boundary violations is highly touted in the field, it is clear though that many supervisors avoid the topic of attraction in therapy. Their discomfort is transmitted to supervisees, who in a behavior paralleling their supervisors, learn to be silent about the topic.

Supervision for this topic will improve when supervisors are comfortable and knowledgeable about the topic, have a clear understanding of the many valid and important reasons why it should be addressed, and have the ability to create a strong alliance with a supervisee in which anxiety provoking and embarrassing topics can be broached.

Conclusions

Mental health professionals know sexual and romantic activity is wrong and consequential. Still it occurs. Thus there is a greater call for an increase in both the number of hours and quality of education, training, and supervision students and professionals receive. Most of the suggestions and recommendations for these enhancements are aspirational and little research has been done in regards to long-term effects. That which exists indicates positive outcomes. There is a consensus that education, training, and supervision are necessary to reduce sexual boundary violations and must begin early in one's career. There is also a consensus that the majority of students, trainees, and supervisees are not receiving adequate or quality education, training, and supervision on this topic.

Summary

- Mental health professionals know sexual and romantic activity is wrong and consequential. Still it occurs. Thus there has been an increasing focus on preventative efforts.
- Education in colleges and universities:
  - The majority of practicing professionals report their formal university training did not prepare them for sexual arousal in the clinical realm.
  - Existing programs are of uncertain quality and have rarely undergone any form of rigorous evaluation.

- o Students may be placed in facilities as part of their internship where unethical practices occur, including sexually questionable behaviors.
- o Training programs should model ethical behavior, be staffed by individuals comfortable with sexual topics, use a variety of approaches to address these topics, focus on increasing self-awareness of risk potential as well as general knowledge about sexual boundary violations, and normalize sexual feelings in treatment.

- Continuing education:

  - o Nearly every jurisdiction that issues a license or certification to practice in the mental health field requires continuing education courses for renewal.
  - o Continuing education programs for sexual boundary violations are of variable quality. Also, there is a lack of agreement as to what a comprehensive training should consist of or how often it should occur.
  - o At present, two themes buttress most available trainings. First, sexual and romantic attraction in clinical settings is normal and to be expected. Second, there are healthy and unhealthy methods of dealing with these feelings.

- Supervision:

  - o Supervision is a crucial ingredient for prevention of boundary violations.
  - o Supervisors and supervisees express reservations about addressing this topic.
  - o Power dynamics in supervisory relationships as well as its evaluative purpose often lead supervisees to elide, lie, or distort their experiences.
  - o Supervision for this topic will improve when supervisors are comfortable and knowledgeable about the topic, have a clear understanding of the many valid and important reasons why it should be addressed, and have the ability to create a strong alliance with a supervisee in which anxiety provoking and embarrassing topics can be broached.

References

Bernsen, A., Tabachnick, B. G., & Pope, K. S. (1994). National survey of social workers' sexual attraction to their clients: Results, implications, and comparison to psychologists. *Ethics & Behavior, 4*(4), 369–388.

Capawana, M. R. (2016). Intimate attractions and sexual misconduct in the therapeutic relationship: Implications for socially just practice. *Cogent Psychology, 3*(1), 1194176.

Celenza, A. (2007). *Sexual boundary violations.* Lanham, MD: Jason Aronson.

Council for Healthcare Regulatory Excellence. (2008). *Learning about sexual boundaries between healthcare professionals and patients: A report on education and training.* London, UK: Author.

Epstein, R. S., & Simon, R. I. (1990). The Exploitation Index: An early warning indicator of boundary violations in psychotherapy. *Menninger Bulletin, 54,* 450–465.

Ford, M. P., & Hendrick, S. S. (2003). Therapists' sexual values for self and clients: Implications for practice and training. *Professional Psychology: Research and Practice, 34*(1), 80.

Fronek, P., Kendall, M., Ungerer, G., Malt, J., Eugarde, E., & Geraghty, T. (2009). Towards healthy professional-client relationships: The value of an interprofessional training course. *Journal of Interprofessional Care, 23*(1), 16–29.

Gabbard, G. O. (1996). Lessons to be learned from the study of sexual boundary violations. *American Journal of Psychotherapy, 50*(3), 311–322.

Gray, L. A., Ladany, N., Walker, J. A., & Ancis, J. R. (2001). Psychotherapy trainees' experience of counterproductive events in supervision. *Journal of Counseling Psychology, 48*(4), 371–383.

Halter, M., Brown, H., & Stone, J. (2007). *Sexual boundary violations by health professionals– An overview of the published empirical literature.* Council for Healthcare Regulatory Excellence.

Hamilton, J. C., & Spruill, J. (1999). Identifying and reducing risk factors related to trainee– Client sexual misconduct. *Professional Psychology: Research and Practice, 30*(3), 318–327.

Housman, L. M., & Stake, J. E. (1999). The current state of sexual ethics training in clinical psychology: Issues of quantity, quality, and effectiveness. *Professional Psychology: Research and Practice, 30*(3), 302.

Ladany, N. (2004). Psychotherapy supervision: What lies beneath. *Psychotherapy Research, 14*(1), 1–19.

Ladany, N. (2007). Does psychotherapy training matter? Maybe not. *Psychotherapy: Theory, Research, Practice, Training, 44,* 392–396.

Ladany, N. (2014). The ingredients of supervisor failure. *Journal of Clinical Psychology, 70*(11), 1094–1103.

Ladany, N., Mori, Y., & Mehr, K. E. (2013). Effective and ineffective supervision. *The Counseling Psychologist, 41*(1), 28–47.

Luca, M., & Boyden, M. (2014). An elephant in the room: A grounded theory of experienced psychotherapists' reactions and attitudes to sexual attraction. In M. Luca (Ed.), *Sexual attraction in therapy: Clinical perspectives on moving beyond the taboo* (pp. 193–208). West Sussex, UK: John Wiley & Sons.

Mehr, K. E., Ladany, N., & Caskie, G. I. (2010). Trainee nondisclosure in supervision: What are they not telling you? *Counselling and Psychotherapy Research, 10*(2), 103–113.

Mehr, K. E., Ladany, N., & Caskie, G. I. (2015). Factors influencing trainee willingness to disclose in supervision. *Training and Education in Professional Psychology, 9*(1), 44–51.

Murray, K. W., & Sommers-Flanagan, J. (2014). Addressing sexual attraction in supervision. In M. Luca (Ed.), *Sexual attraction in therapy: Clinical perspectives on moving beyond the taboo* (pp. 97–114). West Sussex, UK: John Wiley & Sons.

Paxton, C., Lovett, J., & Riggs, M. L. (2001). The nature of professional training and perceptions of adequacy in dealing with sexual feelings in psychotherapy: Experiences of clinical faculty. *Ethics & Behavior, 11*(2), 175–189.

Pope, K. S., & Keith-Spiegel, P. (2008). A practical approach to boundaries in psychotherapy: Making decisions, bypassing blunders, and mending fences. *Journal of Clinical Psychology, 64*(5), 638–652.

Pope, K. S., Keith-Spiegel, P., & Tabachnick, B. G. (2006). Sexual attraction to clients: The human therapist and the (sometimes) inhuman training system. *Training and Education in Professional Psychology, S*(2), 96–111.

Seto, M. C. (1995). Sex with therapy clients: Its prevalence, potential consequences, and implications for psychology training. *Canadian Psychology/Psychologie Canadienne, 36*(1), 70.

Simon, R. I. (1995). The natural history of therapist sexual misconduct: Identification and prevention. *Psychiatric Annals, 25*(2), 90–94.

Steinberg, A. L., & Alpert, J. L. (2017). Sexual boundary violations: An agenda demanding more consideration. *Psychoanalytic Psychology, 34*(2), 221.

Strasburger, L. H., Jorgenson, L., & Sutherland, P. (1992). The prevention of psychotherapist sexual misconduct: Avoiding the slippery slope. *American Journal of Psychotherapy, 46*(4), 544–555.

Tschan, W. (2014). *Professional sexual misconduct in institutions: Causes and consequences, prevention and intervention.* Boston, MA: Hogrefe Publishing.

Vasquez, M. J. (1988). Counselor-client sexual contact: Implications for ethics training. *Journal of Counseling & Development, 67*(4), 238–241.

Organizational Change

10

Sexual boundary violations occur in secret and are difficult to detect. Whether a transgressing professional is actively predatory or an individual caught in the throes of overwhelming emotions, distorted thinking, and driven by unconscious motivations, there is a shared pattern: a purposeful effort to hide what is truly happening with a particular patient. It is impossible for employers to know what is going on behind the closed doors of a mental health provider's office, in their out-of-work interactions, and within contact on private phone calls, texting, and e-mails. What then can an organization do to reduce the risk of a behavior that is purposefully obfuscated and occurs in private? It is clear that current efforts for reducing sexual boundary violations – written policy, reliance on employee's knowledge of ethical requirements and consequences, and, if they occur, trainings in which the behavior is decried – have already had their maximum impact. This chapter posits that additional success will come about when, (1) clinicians recognize that they are on the Boundary Violation Cycle and disclose to a colleague or preferably a supervisor before irreversible damage occurs, and (2) when colleagues and patients report the concerning behavior of a clinician. For these outcomes to become manifest, we must examine organizational functioning. Some organizations will make disclosure – either by the transgressing clinician, a colleague, or a patient – a much safer process than others. Additionally, and far more troubling, organizational practices may implicitly and even explicitly condone boundary crossings and outright violations.

Organizations' Influences on Deviant Behavior

Decades of studies have examined organizational factors that increase or decrease the likelihood that employees will comply with workplace rules and regulations, particularly engagement in what Giacalone and Greenberg (1997) titled "antisocial behavior in organizations" in the first book dedicated to the topic; these include lying, stealing, and sabotage. They acknowledge the machinations of antisocial and even sociopathic individuals in the workplace but find the majority of rule breaking is done by individuals lacking these characteristics. This is true too for sexual harassment in the workplace, including unwanted sexual attention, sexual coercion, and/or misogynistic acts.

Boye and Jones (1997) reviewed several decades of studies to determine which factors related to organizational culture have the most potential to influence behaviors counterproductive to the workplace. First, the authors noted the importance of formal policy for contraindicated behaviors. Second, an organization's record of handling offenders leads employees to draw conclusions as to what would happen to them if they were to engage in the same behavior. The authors conclude that lenient or inconsistent handling of an infraction reinforces the likelihood of future transgressions. Third, oversight and security also reduces risk; individuals are less likely to engage in a contraindicated behavior if there is a high likelihood of detection. Finally, but of no small significance, employees' beliefs about the integrity of an employer influence behavior. A 1995 report (London House & Food Marketing Industry, 1995) determined that ten organizational values were associated with fewer counterproductive behaviors. These were: (1) fairness with employees; (2) caring and empathy; (3) employee empowerment; (4) career-enriching opportunities; (5) equitable pay and benefits; (6) interpersonal cooperation; (7) accurate job–person matching; (8) honesty and ethics; (9) safe working conditions; and (10) job security. Ashforth, Gioia, Robinson, and Trevino (2008), in their review of organization corruption from a systems perspective, conclude employees believe "ethics is not just window dressing but is integrated into daily action" (p. 674). In sum, they determined that those experiencing poor job satisfaction, low perception about an organization's integrity, high certainty that a counterproductive behavior would not be detected, and belief that sanctions would be minimal are more likely to engage in organization antisocial behavior.

Leaders too influence organizational ethics and counterproductive behaviors, and two leadership styles have been highlighted: hostile/abusive leaders and those lacking skills for their position. Tepper (2007) reviewed literature on abusive supervision and lists the following as common displays of this style: petty tyranny; workplace bullying; aggression; undermining; and negative mentoring. Those employees on the receiving end of abusive supervision experience decreased job satisfaction, lowered commitment to an organization, insecurity, diminished feelings of control, and mistrust. In sum, he found that abusive supervision taxes subordinates' coping resources. Other studies find that abusive supervision is correlated with counterproductive organizational behaviors (Duffy, Ganster, & Pagon, 2002; Robinson & Bennett, 1995). Some other leaders are not hostile or abusive but instead appear as disinterested, lacking knowledge, and/or ill equipped for their position. Also, Ashforth et al. (2008) state that leaders who ignore or "turn a blind eye" to unseemly behaviors are not likely to beget trust in subordinates. In contrast, a meta-analysis by Dirks and Ferrin (2002) found that employees' trust in their leaders was associated with many positive behaviors, such as altruism, civic virtue, conscientiousness, courtesy, and sportsmanship.

The influence of colleagues on engagement in counterproductive behaviors is also noted in the literature. Treviño, Weaver, and Reynolds (2006) found that the workplace attitudes and behaviors of peers sway ethical behaviors. Peers not only model what is considered appropriate and inappropriate behavior but also offer approval and disapproval for engagement in these behaviors. Ashforth and Anand (2003), in a well-lauded article, describe the socialization process by which new employees in an organization or a work group incrementally engage in moral compromises and unethical behaviors. While the amorality of certain organizations and fields may attract those with predisposing personality characteristics, it seems that the majority of individuals are gradually socialized into the process; peer influence is of no minor importance during the progression.

A final finding regarding antisocial behaviors in organizations is the influence of stress and frustration; organizations that do not consider the influence of stress on decision-making are perpetuating risk. Peters and O'Connor (1980) compiled a list of the eight most common organizational stressors: (1) job related information; (2) tools and equipment; (3) materials and supplies; (4) budgetary support; (5) required services and help from others; (6) task preparation; (7) time availability; and (8) work environment. While these eight factors apply to all workplaces, other research has targeted stressors associated with employment in a mental health treatment facility, including those treating drug and alcohol-use disorders. Common stressors include poor compensation and benefits, little or no advancement potential, being overburdened, the rapid turn-over of colleagues, lack of administrative support, safety, job security, and the physical environment of the facility (Blankertz & Robinson, 1997; Eby, Burk, & Maher, 2010; Vinokur-Kaplan, Jayaratne, & Chess, 1994). Spector (1997) reminds us that frustration can arise from a singular major event or be the result of cumulative minor frustrations. He then concludes that frustration and stress lead employees to become hostile to rules, act impulsively, to isolate, to be less likely to seek supervision, and to be less likely to report problems.

Sexual Harassment in Organizations

While the above studies examined general antisocial proclivities in organizations, another line of research focuses specifically on sexual harassment in the workplace.

A 2007 meta-analysis of antecedents of workplace sexual harassment determined organizational culture has the largest effect size of any variable in the analysis (Willness, Steel, & Lee, 2007). Several organizational culture factors have been particularly highlighted in the literature. First, general workplace incivility, which is succinctly described by Cortina, Kabat-Farr, Leskinen, Huerta, and Magley (2013) as "rude and discourteous behavior that lacks a clear intent to harm" (p. 1580). Pearson, Andersson, and Porath (2000) offer a more detailed description:

> Workplace civility is behavior that helps to preserve the norms for mutual respect at work; it comprises behaviors that are fundamental to positively connecting with another, building relationships and empathizing. Incivility, in contrast, implies rudeness and disregard toward others. Incivility is mistreatment that may lead to disconnection, breach of relationships and erosion of empathy. Within the work context, incivility entails the violation of workplace norms for mutual respect, such that cooperation and motivation may be hindered broadly.
>
> (p. 125)

Quick and McFadyen (2017), in their review of 20 years of research on the topic, found incivility to be a pivotal organizational factor contributing to sexual harassment as well as mistreatment of racial minorities and LGBT+ individuals. Fitzgerald, Drasgow, Hulin, Gelfand, and Magley (1997) conclude that workplaces communicating tolerance of sexual harassment experience higher levels of this behavior. In particular, Hulin, Fitzgerald, and Drasgow (1996) note that perceived risk to victims for complaining, a lack of sanctions against offenders, and a perception that one's complaints will not be taken seriously are antecedents for sexual harassment.

Summary of Organizational Influences

Decades of research conclude that organizational culture, leadership, and peer interactions are not neutral factors in ethical decision-making. They instead support or detract from formal written policy and the expected standards of a field. In regards to sexual boundary violations, organizational influences occur in three ways:

1. Organizational factors can tax the coping resources of its employees, which can then lead to poor decision-making.
2. Organizational factors can make it less likely an employee will engage in help-seeking behavior from a supervisor. They can also make it less likely colleagues will report concerns about a colleague.
3. Organizations can explicitly or implicitly condone counterproductive behaviors.

Organizational Policy and Change

Organizational practices for reducing counterproductive behavior are consistent in the literature and seven themes are noted:

1. behavioral expectations should be established and clarified, including civility amongst employees;
2. organizations should have written policies and procedures for filing grievances and investigating complaints;
3. leaders should model appropriate behavior;
4. organizations should engage in assessment of its culture by multiple stakeholders and make changes based on feedback;
5. potential employees should be carefully scrutinized in the recruitment and selection process;
6. supervision should occur; and
7. enforcement practices should be in place.

The last theme is particularly powerful. Organizations that ignore, turn a blind eye to, and/or justify behaviors contradicting written policy and expectation are implicitly sanctioning counterproductive behaviors.

At present the onus for sexual boundary violations falls solely on professionals. Organizations can absolve themselves of responsibility for a violation by claiming its employees *should* know better; after all, there are written policies, ethical statements, known consequences, and annual, or possibly even bi-annual, training on this topic. When a violation does occur, organizations can denounce the transgressor as a sociopath or amoral individual who was able to elide otherwise stringent hiring practices. In striking contrast and as reviewed above, decades of research find that organizational factors influence counterproductive behaviors, including unwanted and inappropriate sexual activity. If, as determined by Honig and Barron (2013), boundary violations are an occupational hazard, what should organizations and even respective fields (e.g., psychology, counseling, social work, etc.) be doing to reduce this risk?

A comprehensive policy for reducing sexual boundary violations must prioritize the following goals for employees:

- increasing awareness of their risk;
- teaching self-monitoring and self-assessment;
- seeking supervision as early as possible while in the process of the Boundary Violation Cycle; and
- supporting employees to confront colleagues about alarming behavior and report concerns to administration.

These goals will only be accomplished by normalizing the experience of arousal and attraction in clinical work; preparing employees for arousal and attraction; enhancing supervision; and reducing counterproductive institutional practices.

Normalizing Arousal and Attraction in Clinical Work

Workplaces should not assume new employees have addressed the topic of sexual attraction in clinical work in a thorough manner if at all at any point in their education or careers. As an instructor in a graduate program and trainer on the topic I am ceaselessly astounded as to how many people believe that sexual attraction to a client is wrong and unethical. When attraction occurs – as it will – the involved individuals shamefully hide it. In contrast, and an exemplar in my mind, I witnessed one organization's discussion of the distribution of new patients to available staff. A male counselor reported that one client would be particularly triggering to him at this point in his life. Not only did the client meet some of his arousal templates but also the counselor was in the midst of a "complicated" separation from his long-term romantic partner. This was stated in a group setting surrounded by colleagues and his immediate supervisor. There was no shocked response and the client was simply given to another staff member. The supervisor had made it her goal to normalize sexual feelings in treatment, purposefully ask about these feelings during supervision, show respect when disclosure occurred, and demonstrate willingness and skill in helping her supervisees work through arousal and attraction.

During orientation and throughout their tenure with an organization, employees should be reminded arousal and attraction are common occupational hazards; their presence should be as freely acknowledged as other common hazards, such as burnout. Don't assume that new employees have ever heard this message before.

Preparing Employees for Clinical Arousal and Attraction

Employee training is one of the most common interventions for organizational change and has been a cornerstone for sexual harassment reduction for decades and, even more recently, uncivil and toxic workplaces. Popovich (1988), for example, determined that reduction of sexual harassment in the workplace requires raising employee awareness about sexual harassment, education about its impact on the organization and victim, and explaining reporting procedures. A decade later Williams, Fitzgerald, and Drasgow (1999) found employee education and training is the foundation for organizational sexual harassment efforts. Quick and McFadyen (2017), in their review of 20 years of research on sexual harassment, also support the use of education, particularly offering trainees opportunities to predict and prepare for incidents of sexual harassment. Smith (2018) summarized training efforts in the American Psychological Association's *Monitor on Psychology* and highlighted known best practices, including learning company policy, laws about sexual harassment, expectations for behavior, and procedures for filing complaints; these trainings should be interactive, included multiple delivery methods (e.g., films, role plays, and lectures), assess an understanding of the content, and be offered annually as refresher courses.

While the above studies focus on sexual harassment, others urge that organizations offer training as to expectations for organizational culture. Estes and Wang (2008) promote civility training for all employees (including supervisors). An exemplar of such training is Civility, Respect, and Engagement in the Workplace (CREW), which aims to foster these behaviors in work settings. According to Osatuke, Leiter, Belton, Dyrenforth, and Ramsel (2013), CREW participants define what constitutes a respectful workplace in their particular unit and come to an agreement on which obstacles, including bad habits, get in the way. They then set common goals with respect to civility norms in their workplace. First launched by the United States Veterans Administration, the approach has been used in over a thousand organizations.

Sexual boundary violations specific trainings and preparation for employees are built upon those for sexual harassment and workplace civility. In addition to reinforcing the normalcy of sexual attraction in clinical practice, these trainings will also include:

- practicing a process of ethical decision-making;
- self-care – dealing with others' crises leads to diminished cognitive ability to handle one's own sexual attraction and arousal. Frustration and stress can also lead to impulsivity;
- education about risk potential, particularly ever-changing dynamic risk factors;
- the consequences of sexual boundary violations for professionals, clients, and the organization;
- introduction of the Boundary Violation Cycle and the importance of self-monitoring;
- expected and healthy methods of managing arousal, particularly utilizing the guidance of one's clinical supervisor;
- bystander expectations, which is monitoring by peers for risk status changes or behaviors indicative of boundary crossings by colleagues; and
- a clear description of reporting and enforcement policies, particularly how an allegation of a violation will be handled.

Trainings should be interactive and delivered using various methods, particularly vignettes, role-plays, filmed enactments, and group discussions. The purpose is to expand current didactic training on the topic, which is typically superficial, to a comprehensive approach in which participants explore how they will respond when arousal and attraction do occur. Those facilitating these trainings should approach the topic in a non-shaming and non-judgmental manner and as an occupational hazard which employees have control over.

Finally, as has been recommended for university and military trainings on counterproductive sexual activity, separate trainings for males and females might be considered (e.g., Turchik & Wilson, 2010; Vladutiu, Martin, & Macy, 2011).

Enhanced Supervision

Supervision is another organizational deterrent for sexual boundary violations. We all know from personal experience that there are supervisors whom employees purposefully engage with as little as possible. Ladany (2004) determined supervisors receive little to no training for the position and instead use their own past experiences of supervision as guides for current behavior, which is particularly problematic if this supervision lacked quality. Indeed if an employee determines a supervisor is untrustworthy, unapproachable, indifferent, reactive, or uncomfortable with certain topics they are far less likely to approach them in clinical consultation. For self-disclosure to occur, supervisors must have the ability to create a strong alliance with a supervisee in which anxiety provoking and embarrassing topics can be broached. Subordinates must also recognize that:

- Supervisors normalize the experience of attraction and arousal in clinical work.
- Supervisors are knowledgeable about clinical arousal and attraction, including using it for personal development.
- Supervisors are safe to discuss such concerns.

Healthcare Providers Service Organization and CNA (2019) released a self-assessment for supervisors to evaluate their inclusion of boundary concerns in their work with supervisees. The device is not comprehensive but is instead intended to initiate organization internal discussion and supervisor self-examination. While directed towards counselors, its content is applicable to other disciplines.

Supervisor Self-Assessment

1. I offer appropriate clinical support for counselor supervisees in compliance with supervisory or employment agreements.
2. I educate supervisees about boundary issues, alerting them to the following red flags:
   a. extending the counseling relationship beyond conventional boundaries;
   b. extracting inappropriate fees;
   c. engaging in inappropriate activities with a client;
   d. accepting gifts from or giving gifts to a client;
   e. becoming a business partner with a client; and
   f. connecting inappropriately with a client on a social media site.
3. I conduct ongoing peer review and performance evaluation of all supervisees' competencies, focusing on clinical conduct, ethical awareness, and rapport with colleagues and clients.

4. I am familiar with the provisions of my state's laws governing scope of practice and professional boundaries.
5. I am familiar with the American Counseling Association (ACA) Code of Ethics, in addition to state-specific laws and regulations related to professional conduct and requirements of the relevant licensure/certification/disciplinary board.
6. I inform supervisees of professional and ethical standards and legal responsibilities of the counseling/therapy profession.

Reducing Counterproductive Institutional Practices

While normalizing attraction, training and preparing employees, and enhancing supervision all buttress efforts to reduce sexual boundary violations in mental health treatment facilities, other changes must be considered, including changing counterproductive institutional practices.

Consumer Involvement

While the suggestion of educating consumers about boundaries in therapy has been made for decades, it is rarely implemented. Layman and McNamara (1997) recommend presenting a sexual misconduct brochure to clients entering therapy, which would inform clients of the unethical nature of therapist sexual misbehavior as well as the right to file a complaint. In their study, Thorn, Shealy, and Briggs (1993) found that clients given this literature showed increased ability to understand what is appropriate and inappropriate therapist behavior, see unwanted touch as nontherapeutic, regard a therapist talking a lot about his or her own sex life as inappropriate, view sex in the therapeutic relationship as inappropriate, and to behave assertively within a session if a therapist's behavior should make them feel uncomfortable.

Recall that clients enter treatment with misconceptions about boundaries in treatment often amassed through films and other media. They may also have had questionable treatment experiences in the past and enter work with a new therapist with a misunderstanding of what is appropriate and inappropriate behavior, such as expectations for socializing or contact between sessions. Organizations may choose to proliferate a statement that romantic and sexual relationships between staff and patients are always forbidden due to its detrimental outcome for patients and staff. Others might take a more discreet approach and discuss appropriate boundaries, common boundary concerns, how to manage boundary crossings, and the normalcy of attraction between clients and staff.

Of no minor importance, the knowledge that a client is aware of sexual boundaries and potential legal action may act as an external source of control for clinicians.

Reducing Institutional Avoidance

Administrators rarely learn about sexual boundary violations due to their concealed nature. In many cases though there are subtle hints or suggestions that something is askew. Silence though is a typical response, in spite of the conclusion by Honig and Barron (2013) that for those in the mental health treatment field "boundary violations is a shared occupational hazard" (p. 901). As such we would assume we know how to handle these predicaments. Still Peltz, Gabbard, and COPE (2001) conclude,

> "Many cases of boundary violation never see the light of day because of the extraordinary resistance to recognizing these transgressions within the institutes themselves. As in cases of incest and other family secrets, no one wishes to speak the unspeakable".
>
> (p. 665)

Even when guided by our respective field's ethics, regulatory board directives, and clear institutional policy that such behavior is never appropriate and grounds for dismissal, many individuals do not step forward to report the behavior. Gartrell, Herman, Olarte, Feldstein, and Localio (1987), as a powerful illustration of this problem, surveyed 1423 psychiatrists. 65% reported treating patients who had been sexually involved with previous therapists but only 8% reported these incidents in spite of the majority acknowledging the harm caused to the patient and even supporting mandatory reporting of such incidents.

Obviously one organizational goal is reduction of institutional avoidance. According to Reamer (1992),

> [F]or a profession to be truly self-regulating, it cannot rely entirely on the efforts of dissatisfied or abused clients to file complaints about impaired practitioners. For a variety of reasons, clients often are reluctant to get involved in the formal adjudication process. Therefore,

members of the profession must be vigilant in their efforts to confront the incompetence, unprofessional misconduct, and unethical activities of their colleagues.

(p. 168)

Why doesn't this occur more often? In their work Schoener, Milgrom, Gonsiorek, Luepker, and Conroe (1990) cited the six most common reasons for reluctance to report:

1. lack of belief in the investigatory process;
2. lack of knowledge about complaint alternatives;
3. concerns about the impact on therapy;
4. uncertainty of professional boundaries;
5. concern that an allegation may not bot be true; and
6. fear of retaliation by the alleged offending clinician.

Two decades later Celenza (2007) supported the findings of Schoener and colleagues but found three reasons predominate: fear of retaliation, confusion as to how to respond, and the desire not to hurt a colleague.

Honig and Barron (2013) found that fear of retaliation by the accused in the form of a countersuit directed at the institution or specific employees helps individuals rationalize their inaction. They also report that when a professional transgressor is charismatic and/or influential, colleagues are far more likely to doubt any damaging claims against the person. Slochower (2017), in an article for *Psychoanalytic Psychology*, states fear of being wrong often leads to lack of response:

Frequently, our hands are tied; there's nothing concrete we can do with what we know or suspect. Scared, fearful of making trouble, feeling impotent, we become doubtful. Are we sure? After all, we weren't there. What if we're wrong? Helpless, frustrated, we sideline what we know.

(p. 197)

Others postulate that inaction is often driven by unconscious decision-making. Above-mentioned Slochower (2017) writes that boundary crossings by a colleague lead us to experience anxiety about our own risk for similar behavior; after all, every clinician will experience erotic tension with clients at some point. If my esteemed colleague could engage in this behavior, how likely am I? It is far easier to engage in victim-blaming, splitting, and denial to circumnavigate this anxiety rather than confront our own possible risk.

Finally, aforementioned Peltz and Gabbard (2001) report that violating professionals are advised by their legal representative to deny allegations, and even if litigation is not involved, the risk to one's career and reputation leads transgressors to lie. Celenza (2007) states that the threat to one's character and livelihood is traumatic and that an initial obstructionist approach by the transgressing clinician is to be expected. Still, a trusted colleague's public statements denying culpability places their co-workers in a tense situation: Who should be believed? Maybe the client is lying about the behavior?

While organizations must have a policy for management of sexual boundary violations that takes into account state and county reporting laws, the safety of the involved client, and organizational liability, they too must consider the welfare of the likely terrified and overwhelmed transgressing clinician, who is too often neglected. How do we show compassion to these individuals? How do we help them stop being obstructionist and instead seek help? A policy similar to that for other impaired employees would be a starting point though, of course, a goal of rehabilitation and return to work are topics that remains highly divisive in our associated fields (and will be addressed in the next chapter). A compassionate policy would make it far easier for peers to present their concerns about a colleague to supervisor. Orr (1997) endorses responses that are compassionate, fair, and firm and reminds us that mental health professionals

> are people too, we can let ourselves know that we need not be ashamed, that when we are ill, we may have the same care and attention we provide to others. And we can learn to seek support when we sense vulnerability to a boundary violation and know that, if we do engage in such a violation, we can expect a fair hearing within known guidelines… the ways we treat ourselves and the ways we can constructively manage our vulnerabilities are so essential, not only in the usual ways regarding our own welfare, but because we cannot give more than we have, either to our patients', students', or clients' well-being.
>
> (p. 295)

Celenza (2007) too assumes a compassionate approach when she reminds us, "sexual exploitation in the professional realm is largely unconsciously motivated and multidetermined. Often if involves unresolved narcissistic needs and well as conflicts with authority. Who among us is completely without these?" (p. 145).

Also, organizations' practices – such as turning a blind eye to less serious boundary crossings, hostile and incompetent supervision, workplace incivility, and demonstrating a lack of ethical integrity – need to be targeted, since they make being an informant a most undesirable and even impossible task.

Summary of Organizational Influences

There is no longer any controversy regarding normalizing sexual attraction in clinical practice, preparing clinicians for this attraction, and enhancing supervisors' ability to constructively manage it when it inevitably arises. As such, these three actions are the foundation for a comprehensive plan for minimizing sexual boundary violations in organizations. Another less frequent suggestion is to educate consumers, who often enter treatment with misconceptions about the process, particularly boundaries. Finally, there is a need to consider organizational culture.

Decreasing institutional avoidance while increasing self-disclosure, the best protections against boundary violations from an organizational perspective, necessitates employees believe that an institution will treat them and colleagues in a fair, transparent, and compassionate manner when serious problems occur. Organizations having little integrity, inconsistent policies and practices, are replete with incivility, and/or managed by abusive, disengaged, or incompetent leadership, are inherently unsafe workplaces and will not motivate employees to risk disclosure of their own concerning behaviors and that of colleagues. Also, the confusion following the discovery of a boundary violation, including threatened lawsuits and countersuits, splitting, and shock, often makes a compassionate approach impossible, and this approach is at present an aspiration rather than a reality.

Conclusions

Sexual boundary violations are engaged in furtively, and the very features and dynamics that lead to success in therapy also make violations almost impossible to detect. Current efforts to reduce sexual boundary violations – written policy, reliance on employee's knowledge of ethical requirements, consequences, self-control, and trainings in which the behavior is decried – have already had their maximum impact. There is a need to consider additional preventative practices. The research on workplace deviance in general and sexual harassment specifically offer a way forward. Five suggestions were proffered. The first three, (1) normalizing attraction, (2) comprehensively preparing employees, and (3) enhancing supervision, are widely acknowledged as instrumental for success though their use in actual practice is highly inconsistent. Another common suggestion, (4) consumer education, could be an adjunct to the above practices but too is rarely used. Finally, (5) fostering organizational practices that counter institutional avoidance, particularly civility, fairness, consistency, adherence to ethics, transparency, and compassion. The combination of the above offers the best pathway to reducing institutional avoidance and increasing self-disclosure, which are essential to recognition and detection of transgressing clinicians.

Summary

- Sexual boundary violations are purposefully concealed and detection is problematic due to the privacy characteristics inherent in therapy.
- Current efforts for reducing sexual boundary violations in clinical practice have already had their maximum impact.
- The two best methods for learning of a boundary transgression are self-disclosure and colleague/co-worker reporting concerns.
- Colleagues often ignore hints or suggestions that a co-worker is engaged in boundary crossings or violations. Also, fear of retaliation, confusion as to how to respond, and the desire not to hurt their colleague lead professionals to remain silent about concerning behaviors.
- Organizational factors such as culture, leadership, and peers influence the prevalence of sexual boundary violations as well as institutional avoidance.
- A comprehensive policy for reducing sexual boundary violations must prioritize the following goals for employees:
  - increasing awareness of their risk;
  - teaching self-monitoring and self-assessment;
  - seeking supervision as early as possible while in the process of the Boundary Violation Cycle; and
  - supporting employees to confront colleagues about alarming behavior and report concerns to administration.

- The above goals will be accomplished via:

    o normalizing sexual attraction in clinical practice;

    o training clinicians to prepare for arousal and attraction in clinical practice;

    o enhancing supervisors' ability to constructively work with the supervisees' attraction and arousal;

    o educating consumers, who often enter treatment with misconceptions about the process, particularly boundary issues; and

    o fostering organizational practices that counter institutional avoidance, particulalry civility, fairness, consistency, adherence to ethics, transparency, and compassion.

References

Ashforth, B. E., & Anand, V. (2003). The normalization of corruption in organizations. In R. M. Kramer & B. M. Staw (Eds.), *Research in organizational behavior* (pp. 1–52). Oxford: Elsevier.

Ashforth, B. E., Gioia, D. A., Robinson, S. L., & Trevino, L. K. (2008). Re-viewing organizational corruption. *Academy of Management Review, 33*(3), 670–684.

Blankertz, L.E. & Robinson, S.E. (1997). Turnover intentions of community mental health workers in psychosocial rehabilitation services. *Community Mental Health Journal, 33*(6), 517–529.

Boye, M.W., & Jones, J. W. (1997). Organizational culture and employee counterproductivity. In R.A. Giacalone & J. Greenberg (Eds.), *Antisocial behaviors in organizations* (pp. 172–184). Thousand Oaks, CA: Sage.

Celenza, A. (2007). *Sexual boundary violations*. Lanham, MD: Jason Aronson.

Cortina, L. M., Kabat-Farr, D., Leskinen, E. A., Huerta, M., & Magley, V. J. (2013). Selective incivility as modern discrimination in organizations: Evidence and impact. *Journal of Management, 39*(6), 1579–1605.

Dirks, K. T., & Ferrin, D. L. (2002). Trust in leadership: Meta-analytic findings and implications for research and practice. *Journal of Applied Psychology, 87*(4), 611–628.

Duffy, M. K., Ganster, D. C., & Pagon, M. (2002). Social undermining in the workplace. *Academy of Management Journal, 45*(2), 331–351.

Eby, L. T., Burk, H., & Maher, C. P. (2010). How serious of a problem is staff turnover in substance abuse treatment? A longitudinal study of actual turnover. *Journal of Substance Abuse Treatment, 39*(3), 264–271.

Estes, B., & Wang, J. (2008). Integrative literature review: Workplace incivility: Impacts on individual and organizational performance. *Human Resource Development Review, 7*(2), 218–240.

Fitzgerald, L. F., Drasgow, F., Hulin, C. L., Gelfand, M. J., & Magley, V. J. (1997). Antecedents and consequences of sexual harassment in organizations: A test of an integrated model. *Journal of Applied Psychology, 82*(4), 578–589.

Gartrell, N., Herman, J., Olarte, S., Feldstein, M., & Localio, R. (1987). Reporting practices of psychiatrists who knew of sexual misconduct by colleagues. *American Journal of Orthopsychiatry, 57*(2), 287–295.

Giacalone, R.A., & Greenberg, J. (1997). *Antisocial behaviors in organizations.* Thousand Oaks, CA: Sage.

Healthcare Providers Service Organization & CNA. (2019). *Counselor spotlight: Boundaries.* Fort Washington, PA: Author.

Honig, R. G., & Barron, J. W. (2013). Restoring institutional integrity in the wake of sexual boundary violations: A case study. *Journal of the American Psychoanalytic Association, 61*(5), 897–924.

Hulin, C. L., Fitzgerald, L. F., & Drasgow, F. (1996). Organizational influences on sexual harassment. In M. S. Stockdale (Ed.), *Sexual harassment in the workplace: Perspectives, frontiers, and response strategies, women and work: A research and policy series* (Vol. 5, pp. 127–150). Thousand Oaks, CA: Sage Publications.

Ladany, N. (2004). Psychotherapy supervision: What lies beneath. *Psychotherapy Research, 14*(1), 1–19.

Layman, M. J., & McNamara, J. R. (1997). Remediation for ethics violations: Focus on psychotherapists' sexual contact with clients. *Professional Psychology: Research and Practice, 28*(3), 281–292.

London House & Food Marketing Industry. (1995). *Fifth annual report of supermarket employee behavior.* Rosemont, IL: London House.

Orr, P. (1997). Psychology impaired? *Professional Psychology: Research and Practice, 28*(3), 293–296.

Osatuke, K., Leiter, M., Belton, L., Dyrenforth, S., & Ramsel, D. (2013). Civility, Respect and Engagement at the Workplace (CREW): A national organization development program at the Department of Veterans Affairs. *Journal of Management Policies and Practices, 1*(2), 25–34.

Pearson, C. M., Andersson, L. M., & Porath, C. L. (2000). Assessing and attacking workplace incivility. *Organizational Dynamics, 29*(2), 123–137.

Peltz, M. L., Gabbard, G. O., & COPE Group on Boundary Violations. (2001). Speaking the unspeakable: Institutional reactions to boundary violations by training analysts. *Journal of the American Psychoanalytic Association, 49*(2), 659–673.

Peters, L. H., & O'Connor, E. J. (1980). Situational constraints and work outcomes: The influences of a frequently overlooked construct. *Academy of Management Review, 5*(3), 391–397.

Popovich, P. M. (1988). Sexual harassment in organizations. *Employee Responsibilities and Rights Journal, 1*(4), 273–282.

Quick, J. C., & McFadyen, M. (2017). Sexual harassment: Have we made any progress? *Journal of Occupational Health Psychology, 22*(3), 286–298.

Reamer, F. G. (1992). The impaired social worker. *Social Work, 37*(2), 165–170.

Robinson, S. L., & Bennett, R. J. (1995). A typology of deviant workplace behaviors: A multidimensional scaling study. *Academy of Management Journal, 38*(2), 555–572.

Schoener, G. R., Milgrom, J. H., Gonsiorek, J. C., Luepker, E. T., & Conroe, R. M. (1990). *Psychotherapists' sexual involvement with clients: Intervention and prevention.* Minneapolis, MN: Walk-in Counseling Ctr.

Slochower, J. (2017). Don't tell anyone. *Psychoanalytic Psychology, 34*(2), 195–200.

Smith, B. L. (2018). What it really takes to stop sexual harassment. *Monitor on Psychology, 49*(2), 36–40.

Spector, P. E. (1997). The role of frustration in antisocial behavior at work. In R. A. Giacalone & J. Greenberg (Eds.), *Antisocial behaviors in organizations* (pp. 1–17). Thousand Oaks, CA: Sage.

Tepper, B. J. (2007). Abusive supervision in work organizations: Review, synthesis, and research agenda. *Journal of Management, 33*(3), 261–289.

Thorn, B. E., Shealy, R. C., & Briggs, S. D. (1993). Sexual misconduct in psychotherapy: Reactions to a consumer-oriented brochure. *Professional Psychology: Research and Practice, 24*(1), 75–82.

Treviño, L. K., Weaver, G. R., & Reynolds, S. J. (2006). Behavioral ethics in organizations: A review. *Journal of Management, 32*(6), 951–990.

Turchik, J. A., & Wilson, S. M. (2010). Sexual assault in the US military: A review of the literature and recommendations for the future. *Aggression and Violent Behavior, 15*(4), 267–277.

Vinokur-Kaplan, D., Jayaratne, S., & Chess, W. A. (1994). Job satisfaction and retention of social workers in public agencies, non-profit agencies, and private practice: The impact of workplace conditions and motivators. *Administration in Social Work, 18*(3), 93–121.

Vladutiu, C. J., Martin, S. L., & Macy, R. J. (2011). College-or university-based sexual assault prevention programs: A review of program outcomes, characteristics, and recommendations. *Trauma, Violence, & Abuse, 12*(2), 67–86.

Williams, J. H., Fitzgerald, L. F., & Drasgow, F. (1999). The effects of organizational practices on sexual harassment and individual outcomes in the military. *Military Psychology, 11*(3), 303–328.

Willness, C. R., Steel, P., & Lee, K. (2007). A meta-analysis of the antecedents and consequences of workplace sexual harassment. *Personnel Psychology, 60*(1), 127–162.

Removal or
Rehabilitation

11

Professionals engaging in sexual boundary violations can self-report to colleagues, supervisors, the agencies in which they work, and to licensing and certification boards. Should these individuals be allowed to ever practice again? Pope (1994), in his groundbreaking and seminal work on sexual boundary violations, concludes they should not be given this opportunity. Ryan (2012) questions though whether a hard-line policy is the best course of action; he instead promotes one that examines the subtleties of each individual case with compassion before determining consequences. Canaris (2003), in a similar vein states,

> Certainly I have encountered frankly predatory professionals whose risk of breaching boundaries is very high no matter what is done for them. I have also encountered many whose compulsive offending arises from long unrecognized disorders of mood and anxiety. For these people, Axis II issues are often an important part of the picture, either in the context of personality disorder or the accentuation of personality traits by primary psychiatric illness... However, merely casting out the bad apples does not sweeten the barrel or make our community safer... it allows us as a professional community to deny the potential within each and every one of us to breach boundaries.
>
> (p. 407)

Rehabilitation Protocols

While many offending professionals, such as those of a predatory nature or with personality disorders, need to be removed from the field, others can be taught to safely practice again, even if this requires modifications in their practice. Layman and McNamara (1997) describe a litany of remediation approaches, including education and training, particularly for ethical issues; an informal support network for impaired professionals in which members could reach out to one another during stressful or high-risk situations; practice oversight, including periodic review by supervisors and colleagues; practice limitations, in which a transgressing clinicians are curtailed from working with specific patients (e.g., a professional who engaged in a boundary violation with a female may only be allowed to work with males); and mandated personal therapy. They also suggest alerting clients beforehand that the professionals they are about to work with have a history of a sexual boundary violation. This latter approach too is promoted by Strasburger, Jorgenson, and Sutherland (1992), who state that patients have the right to knowledge of risk so they can make an informed choice. Brown (1997) highlights the importance of victim feedback in the rehabilitation process, which is often ignored. She suggests that offending professionals apologize to victims, listen to and acknowledge the pain, anger, and betrayal that occurred, and affirm that the latter were not in any way responsible for the behavior. The author also attests that sexual boundary crossings result in collateral victims, particularly colleagues, who also feel aghast and betrayed. Too often the transgressing clinician is terminated and disappears completely from their lives. Rehabilitation thus should also include the opportunity for the offender and colleagues to meet to discuss the impact a violation has had on all involved.

Schoener and Gonsiorek (1988) describe a model of assessment and rehabilitation planning based on their work with over 1000 mental health workers who had engaged in sexual boundary violations. Assessment considers the following data: descriptions of all offenses; presence or absence of psychopathology; practice style, particularly as they relate to professional boundaries; practice setting, including presence of supervision; nature of clientele served, including the demographic with which boundary violations occurred; and miscellaneous factors, such as significant life events or particular issues that were triggered by a client. This data is collected through interviews with the professional as well as collateral sources such as supervisors, colleagues, and even family. Using this data, the researchers formulate a hypothesis of causality, or in their words, a "configural interpretation of a number of observations" (p. 230). A rehabilitation plan is developed, much of which was described in above-mentioned Layman and McNamara (1997). In addition, they support changes in therapy style, typically becoming more conservative in self-disclosure and physical contact of any kind. Also, existing organizational practices may need to be modified or the practitioner would be required to move to another agency that has clearer polices and standards as well as improved supervision. Finally, Schoener and Gonsiorek (1988), acknowledging that rehabilitation cannot be achieved for some predatory individuals, support vocational counseling to assist them to transition into new non-therapy fields.

Gartrell, Herman, Olarte, Feldstein, and Localio (1988) also present an overview of rehabilitation with "sexually exploitative therapists" in their work with the Walk-In Counseling Center, an agency dedicated to development of strategies to manage and reduce sexual exploitation in the mental health field. They too begin with a thorough assessment, including interviewing collateral sources and obtaining records such as reports of other misconduct, supervisory evaluations, records of training, and past mental health treatment. Additional psychological testing may be required. Based on these above sources, a diagnostic formulation is proffered as well as a rehabilitation plan. In the case of predatory clinicians, it is advised they change careers. For others, personal psychotherapy, enhanced supervision, and practice limitations (e.g., only engaging in group therapy or treating patients of one gender) are typical recommendations. Supervisors and regulatory agencies monitor the plan.

Tschan (2014) describes a semi-structured, manual-based, boundary-training rehabilitation program consisting of 24 modules and lasting a minimum of 2 years for professionals engaging in boundary violations as a requisite for returning to the field. The goals of this training are to help professionals take responsibility for their behavior, learn how to maintain boundaries, and, of the greatest importance, prevent future offending. Those presenting with co-occurring disorders must engage in treatment for these conditions prior to boundary training. As with the aforementioned models, the rehabilitation process begins with a thorough assessment, the development of a treatment plan, engagement in boundary training, and job re-entry, along with careful monitoring by at least one colleague who offers feedback and concerns to the offending professional's treatment provider. This protocol mandates homework assignments, including watching specific films, bibliotherapy (reading and discussing papers), and formulation of an apology letter to victim(s) which is not sent due to risk of re-traumatization but that nevertheless demonstrates empathic awareness on the part of the professional of the impact of the boundary violation. Tschan's protocol explores topics such as:

- the client–professional relationship;
- boundaries;
- epidemiology of sexual violations;
- trauma;

- survivors' healing journey;
- fantasies;
- relapse prevention; and
- responsibility.

Jorgenson (1995) expressed concerns about rehabilitation efforts due to the number of liability issues arise that arise. For example, if a rehabilitated professional engages in another boundary violation, the rehabilitation provider may be liable for failure to provide proper treatment. Subsequent employers may also be liable for negligently hiring or retaining an abusive therapist; they could also be held liable for negligent supervision of employees. Though Jorgenson described steps employers can undertake to limit exposure to liability, particularly rigorous monitoring, patient and colleague feedback, reports from a transgressor's therapist, and practice limitations, she still cautions these may not be enough to shield against direct liability for negligent hiring, retention, and supervision. Thus professionals undergoing rehabilitation find themselves in a double bind. They cannot find agencies willing to risk working with them thus pushing them into private practice, which then limits supervision and colleague input, two necessary components for successful rehabilitation.

One final recommendation is the use of polygraphs (commonly referred to as lie detector tests). Though their use in sex offender treatment remains contentious, a number of studies and reviews have found value in them (e.g., English, Jones, Pasini-Hill, Patrick, & Cooley-Towell, 2000; Grubin, 2008; Kokish, Levenson, & Blasingame, 2005). Maintenance or monitoring polygraphs verify whether an offender is complying with the terms and stipulations of his supervision; its assists in both detecting reoffending if it occurs and acting as a deterrent. A rehabilitation plan for professionals may require an annual polygraph or one of even more frequency.

The rehabilitation process, including assessment, therapy, and polygraph will cost no small amount, and it is certain that many mental health workers will not be able to afford it. This too is a question that will need to be addressed.

Summary of Rehabilitation

Rehabilitation of professionals engaging in boundary violations at a minimum consists of a thorough assessment, mandated therapy for the transgressing professional, augmented supervision, and practice limitations. Additional preventative tools are education and training, support groups, patient notification, victim amends, and polygraphs.

Rehabilitation, however comprehensive and individualized, remains an extremely contentious topic. Some decry any such efforts claiming that rehabilitation remains under-researched and that the population is simply at too high risk to safely engage in practice. Others though, while acknowledging the intractability of predatory offenders and those with personality disorders, propose that many others can safely return to work, even if this requires possible lifelong limitations. Orr (1997), for example, writes,

> [B]oundary violators are on a continuum regarding rehabilitation potential, that some persons can be successfully rehabilitated and others cannot. I can personally confirm the dimensions of the continuum, having had experience with a successfully rehabilitated colleague as well as with those who have proven to be nonrehabilitative. We need to learn much more about the continuum.
>
> (p. 295)

Unfortunately, due to the unwillingness of agencies and organizations to hire these individuals and the costs of participating in rehabilitation, few undergo the process, thus limiting our knowledge of its actual success.

Conclusions

Rehabilitation of transgressing professionals has been in use for decades, and it has many proponents. While it is contraindicated for predatory individuals and those with personality disorders, who are best served by assisting them to find different fields in which to work, rehabilitation can be successful for others. Obstacles include pragmatic concerns, such as cost, liability issues, and unwillingness by employers to hire rehabilitated professionals. A more profound concern is the use of polarized "us and them" and "splitting" occurring in the field, which depicts boundary-transgressing professionals as irredeemable. The reality is that all clinicians are capable of a boundary violation dependent on proximal and distal risk factors and changing life circumstances. Do we forever shun a transgressing mental health professional or carefully allow them back in the field after a period of punishment and rehabilitation? The field offers no consensus on this question.

Summary

- Professionals engaging in boundary violations can self-report to colleagues, supervisors, the agencies in which they work, and to licensing and certification boards.
- Rehabilitation of offending clinicians is a controversial topic in the field.
- While many offending professionals, such as those of a predatory nature or with personality disorders, need to be removed from the field, others can be taught to safely practice again.
- Rehabilitation of professionals engaging in boundary violations at a minimum consists of a thorough assessment, mandated therapy for the transgressing professional, augmented supervision, and practice limitations. Additional preventative tools are education and training, support groups, patient notification, victim amends, and polygraphs.

References

Brown, L. S. (1997). Remediation, amends, or denial? *Professional Psychology: Research and Practice, 28*(3), 297–299.

Canaris, C. (2003). The 'out of house'solution to boundary violations. *Australasian Psychiatry, 11*(4), 406–409.

English, K., Jones, L., Pasini-Hill, D., Patrick, D., & Cooley-Towell, S. (2000). The value of polygraph testing in sex offender management. *Colorado Department of Public Safety.*

Gartrell, N., Herman, J. L., Olarte, S., Feldstein, M., & Localio, R. (1988). Management and rehabilitation of sexually exploitive therapists. *Psychiatric Services, 39*(10), 1070–1074.

Grubin, D. (2008). The case for polygraph testing of sex offenders. *Legal and Criminological Psychology, 13*(2), 177–189.

Jorgenson, L. M. (1995). Rehabilitating sexually exploitative therapists: A risk management perspective. *Psychiatric Annals, 25*(2), 118–122.

Kokish, R., Levenson, J. S., & Blasingame, G. D. (2005). Post-conviction sex offender polygraph examination: Client-reported perceptions of utility and accuracy. *Sexual Abuse: A Journal of Research and Treatment, 17*(2), 211–221.

Layman, M. J., & McNamara, J. R. (1997). Remediation for ethics violations: Focus on psychotherapists' sexual contact with clients. *Professional Psychology: Research and Practice, 28*(3), 281–292.

Orr, P. (1997). Psychology impaired? *Professional Psychology: Research and Practice, 28*(3), 293–296.

Pope, K. S. (1994). *Sexual involvement with therapists.* Washington, DC: American Psychological Association.

Ryan, C. J. (2012). An unethical policy on sexual boundary violations. *Australian and New Zealand Journal of Psychiatry, 46,* 584.

Schoener, G. R., & Gonsiorek, J. (1988). Assessment and development of rehabilitation plans for counselors who have sexually exploited their clients. *Journal of Counseling & Development, 67*(4), 227–232.

Strasburger, L. H., Jorgenson, L., & Sutherland, P. (1992). The prevention of psychotherapist sexual misconduct: Avoiding the slippery slope. *American Journal of Psychotherapy, 46*(4), 544–555.

Tschan, W. (2014). *Professional sexual misconduct in institutions: Causes and consequences, prevention and intervention.* Boston: Hogrefe Publishing.

Conclusion

We're All in This Together

The most effectual intervention for decreasing sexual boundary violations in mental health practice is clinician self-monitoring for sexual arousal and romantic attraction towards clients, and seeking supervision or peer consultation promptly when it is recognized. The longer the delay in seeking guidance – likely due to embarrassment or overconfidence in self-management ability – the more likely one is to progress ever closer to a violation.

While the above suggestion is sound and certainly attainable it nevertheless risks keeping us stranded in the same quagmire of blame occurring today. Licensing and certification boards, professional associations, and employers denounce transgressing clinicians as lacking self-control, sociopathic, and even predatory, which absolves these former entities of any responsibility; after all, they reason, professionals know this behavior is wrong and shouldn't do it. Using this conceptualization of the problem, it is the duty of mental health workers and them alone to monitor for arousal and seek help when it occurs; no systemic change is needed except possibly to increase consequences to the point that no sane or reasonable person would even think of acting on attraction to a client. The problem is that attraction, particularly of a sexual nature, plays havoc with our reasoning abilities. This book has made it clear that a host of insidious unconscious influences and distorted thinking lead far too many mental health workers to sexual activity with clients in spite of known risks, no matter how catastrophic.

The above effectual remedy needs to be buttressed with supports from all who have a stake in resolving this ongoing crisis. The first crucial step is acknowledging that, without doubt, sexual boundary violations are an occupational hazard; they are not typically the end result of predatory clinicians or poor hiring decisions. They are instead an inevitable and unavoidable risk arising when two human beings, each with their own fragilities, come into contact with each other to discuss profound and often-intimate matters in privacy. This occupational hazard seems particularly challenging for male clinicians to navigate as evinced by the gender discrepancies found in every examination of the topic. Thus an accurate reframing of sexual boundary violations is not that they are the willful acts of dissolute clinicians but rather an unfortunate outcome for those who do not have the support needed to traverse a common occupational hazard.

Learning to manage this risk is a process that must begin in the formative years of mental health workers. Most university and college programs offer minimal education on sexual topics in general and even less on management of one's own attraction and arousal. These are topics that should be introduced early and continually reinforced. So too should the normalcy of sexual attraction in clinical practice. Employers too have a significant part to play, and this entails more than disseminating policy stating sexual boundary violations are unacceptable. They should remind employees that sexual attraction towards and from clients is to be expected and that there is nothing inherently wrong with these human responses. They should also make a policy known that attraction needs to be addressed with a supervisor. Still, the two most important preventative measures employers can take are: (1) an assessment of the workplace culture for those influences promoting counterproductive behaviors and making changes based on the results; and (2) hiring and training supervisors who are knowledgeable about the occupational hazard of sexual boundary violations; these supervisors will be able to safely and reassuringly guide supervisees in working through sexual attraction without eliciting shame or fear. A lack of supervisors or colleagues who can handle the topic of sexual attraction in clinical work will preclude professionals from seeking guidance when arousal occurs, which we know is essential for reducing boundary violations. But, at present, lack of quality supervisors, particularly for sexual topics, is the reality of the field.

Finally, licensing and certification agencies as well as professional associations must admit that their efforts at prevention have achieved maximum gains. Having members sign an ethics statement condemning sexual boundary violations has not and will not end the behavior. This too will be the same outcome of escalating professional consequences for violators, which will only make transgressors more diligent in obfuscating the behavior and lead to desperate measures when a violation is discovered, including suicide attempts. Instead, these entities should support augmented efforts by universities and employers, persistently and deliberately highlight the occupational hazard of sexual boundary violations, and demand thorough training on the topic instead of its typically cursory inclusion in general ethics or dual relationships trainings. They can also lead the way in examining the feasibility of a rehabilitation process.

Presently there is an unfortunate and mistaken consensus that the mental health field has done all it can to reduce sexual boundary violations. This subsumes an often implicit belief that it is now solely up to clinicians to guard against them. While this book does support the contention that it is indeed imperative for clinicians to engage in self-monitoring, it also highlights the findings that colleges and universities, employers, licensing and certification agencies, and professional associations can do much, much more to assist professionals in learning to recognize risk, engage in self-monitoring, and seek supervision and consultation. Professionals must do more but so too must all those who support them to engage in a career that unfortunately comes with an occupational hazard of sexual boundary violations.

Index

For Product Safety Concerns and Information please contact our EU
representative GPSR@taylorandfrancis.com
Taylor & Francis Verlag GmbH, Kaufingerstraße 24, 80331 München, Germany